THE NEUROTIC CONSTITUTION

THE
NEUROTIC CONSTITUTION

OUTLINES OF A COMPARATIVE INDIVIDUAL-
ISTIC PSYCHOLOGY AND PSYCHOTHERAPY

BY

DR. ALFRED ADLER

AUTHORIZED ENGLISH TRANSLATION

By

BERNARD GLUECK

and

JOHN E. LIND

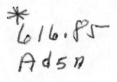

BOOKS FOR LIBRARIES PRESS
FREEPORT, NEW YORK

First Published 1926
Reprinted 1972

Library of Congress Cataloging in Publication Data

Adler, Alfred, 1870-1937.
  The neurotic constitution.

  ([BCL/select bibliographies reprint series])
  Reprint of the 1926 ed., which is a translation of
Uber den nervösen charakter.
  Bibliography: p.
  1. Neuroses. I. Title.
RC530.A3213 1972   616.85   74-39684
ISBN 0-8369-9925-8

PRINTED IN THE UNITED STATES OF AMERICA
BY
NEW WORLD BOOK MANUFACTURING CO., INC.
HALLANDALE, FLORIDA 33009

PREFACE

After I had made the attempt to investigate in the "Studie über Minderwertigkeit von Organen," the structure and tectonic of organs in association with their genetic basis, their functional capability and destiny, I proceeded, supporting myself upon already available data as well as upon my own experience, to apply the same method in the study of psychopathology. In the book before us are embraced the most important results of my comparative, individual-psychologic studies of the neuroses.

As was the case in the theory of somatic inferiority, an empiric basis is made use of in comparative individual-psychology for the purpose of establishing a fictive standard of normality in order to enable one to measure and compare with it grades of deviation from it. In both of these scientific endeavors, the comparative method of study reckons with the origin of phenomena, dismisses from consideration the present and seeks to outline from them the future. This method of approach leads us to view the compulsion of evolution and the pathological elaboration as the result of a conflict which breaks forth in the organic sphere for the purpose of attaining equipoise, functional capability and adaptation; the same struggle in the psychic sphere is under the command of a fictitious idea of personality whose influence dominates the development of the neurotic character and symptoms. If in the organic sphere, "the individual develops into a unit mass in which all of the individual parts cooperate toward a common goal" (Virchow), if the various abilities and tendencies of the individual tend toward a purposefully directed, unit-personality, then we may look upon every single manifestation of life as if in its past, present and future there are contained traces of a dominating, guiding idea.

In this way it has appeared to the author of this book, that the most minute trait of psychic life is permeated by a purpose-force. Comparative, individualistic psychology sees in every psychic event the impress, so to speak, or symbol of a uniformly directed plan of life which only comes more clearly to light in the neuroses and psychoses.

The result of such an investigation of the neurotic character should furnish proof of the value and utility of our method of comparative, individualistic psychology in the problems of mental life.   THE AUTHOR.
Vienna, February, 1912.

INTRODUCTION

"Omnia ex opinione suspensa sunt: non ambitio tantum ad illam respicit et luxuria et avaricia. Ad opinionem dolemus. Tam miser est quisque, quam credidit."

SENECA, *Epist*. 78, 13.

The study of the neurotic character is an essential part of neuro-psychology. Like all other psychic phenomena it can only be understood when taken in connection with the entire psychic life. A cursory knowledge of the neuroses suffices to enable one to discover that which is peculiarly characteristic in them and all writers who have studied the problem of nervousness have laid particular stress upon certain peculiar traits of character. The opinion was a general one that the neurotic shows a series of sharply emphasized traits of character which exceed the normal standard. The marked sensitiveness, the irritable debility, the suggestibility, the egotism, the penchant for the fantastic, the estrangement from reality, but also more special traits such as tyranny, malevolence, a self-sacrificing virtue, coquetry, anxiety and absent-mindedness

are met with in the majority of case histories and
it would be necessary to detail all writers who
have thoroughly studied the subject in order to
endorse their contributions. Of the more recent
ones, Janet, who has carried on the traditions of
the famous French school and who has brought
to light some very important and ingenious
analyses, must be especially mentioned. His
emphasis of the neurotic's "sentiment d'incomple-
tude" particularly, is so wholly in harmony with
the results offered by me that I am justified in
seeing in my work an extension of this most important fundamental fact of the mental life of the
neurotic.

No matter where one begins with the analysis
of psychogenic disorders, one and the same phenomenon forces itself upon one's attention after
the briefest observation, namely, that the entire
picture of the neurosis as well as all its symptoms
are influenced by, nay, even wholly provoked by
an imaginary fictitious goal. This final purpose
has a creative, directive and adjustive power.
The potency of this "goal idea" is revealed to us
by the trend and evaluation of the pathological
phenomena and should one attempt to dispense
with this assumption there remains nothing but a
confusing mass of impulses, trends, components,
debilities and anomalies which has made the obscurity of the neurosis impenetrable to some, while

others have undertaken bold exploratory journeys into this field.

Pierre Janet has certainly recognized this relationship as is shown in his classical descriptions of the "Hysterical Psyche," 1894,[1] but he avoided a detailed description. He expressly maintains, "I have until now only described general and simple traits of character which by means of their association and under the influence of definite extraneous circumstances may produce all kinds of curious behavior and conduct." It is entirely out of place here to enter into a detailed discussion of Janet's description for this treatise would then resemble more a moral romance than a clinical study. Having adhered to this attitude even up to his latest contributions on the subject, Janet, notwithstanding his keen insight into the relationship between the psychology of the neuroses and moral philosophy, never entered the road to synthesis.

It remained for Joseph Breuer, a man well versed in current German philosophy, to discover the gem which lay in his path. He directed his attention to the meaning of the symptoms and undertook to ascertain the source and purpose of the same from the only one who could give them —from the patient. In so doing the author founded a method which seeks to explain indi-

[1] Translated by Dr. Max Kahane.

vidual psychological phenomena historically and genetically with the assistance of a preliminary hypothesis, i.e., that of the determinism of psychic phenomena. The manner in which this method has been extended and improved upon by Sigmund Freud with the host of problems and attempted solutions therewith connected belongs to contemporaneous history and has met with both recognition and contradiction. Less for the purpose of following a critical bent than for the purpose of making clear my own position I beg leave to separate from the fruitful and valuable contributions of Freud three of his fundamental views as erroneous inasmuch as they threaten to impede progress in the understanding of the neuroses. The first objection is directed against the view that the libido is the motive force behind the phenomena of the neurosis. On the contrary it is the neurosis which shows more clearly than does normal psychic conduct how by means of this neurotic positing of a "final purpose," the apperception of pleasure, its selection and power are all driven in the direction of this final purpose so that the neurotic can really only follow the allurement of the acquisition of pleasure with his healthy psychic force, so to speak, while for the neurotic portion only "higher" goals are of value.

The neurotic goal (Zwecksetzung) has revealed itself to us in the heightened ego-consciousness (Persönlichkeitsgefühl) whose simplest formula is to be recognized in an exaggerated "masculine protest" (Männlichen Protest). This formula: "I wish to be a complete man" is the guiding fiction in every neurosis, claiming higher reality values than even the normal psyche. The libido, the sex-impulses and the tendencies to sexual perversions arrange themselves in accordance with this guiding principle, no matter whence they originate. Nietzsche's "Will to power" and "Will to seem" embrace many of our views, which again resemble in some respects the views of Féré and the older writers, according to whom the sensation of pleasure originates in a feeling of power, that of pain in a feeling of feebleness (Ohnmacht).

A second objection is directed against Freud's fundamental view of the sexual etiology of the neuroses, a view which Pierre Janet approached very closely when he asked, "Is sexual feeling then the center around which all other psychological syntheses are built up?" The applicability of the sexual picture deceives the normal person and especially the neurotic. But it must not deceive the psychologist. The sexual content in the neurotic phenomenon originates primarily in the imaginary antithesis: "Masculine-feminine" and is evolved through a change of form of the "masculine protest." The sexual trend in the fantasy

and life of the neurotic follows the direction of
the "masculine goal," and is really not a trend,
but a compulsion. The whole picture of the
sexual neurosis is nothing more than a portrait
depicting the distance which the patient is removed from the imaginary masculine goal and the
manner in which he seeks to bridge it. It is
strange that Freud, a skillful connoisseur of the
symbolic in life, was not able to discover the symbolic in "sexual apperception," to recognize the
sexual as a jargon, a *modus dicendi*. But we can
understand this when we take into consideration
the more extensive basic error, i.e., the assumption
that the neurotic is under the influence of infantile wishes, which come to life nightly (Dream
theory) as well as in connection with certain occasions in life. In reality these infantile wishes
already stand under the compulsion of the imaginary goal and themselves usually bear the character of a guiding thought suitably arrayed, and
adapt themselves to symbolic expression purely
for reasons of thought economy. A sickly girl
who during her entire childhood in her consciousness of an unusual insecurity leans upon her
father and in so doing strives to become superior
to her mother, may comprehend this psychic constellation in the form of an incest, as if she wished
to be the wife of her father. Thereby the goal
is both attained and effective; her insecurity is

only abolished when she is with her father. Her developed psycho-motor intelligence, her unconsciously active memory combats all feelings of uncertainty with the same aggression, with the adequate expedient, to take refuge in the father as if she were his wife. There she finds that heightened ego-consciousness which she has set for her goal, which she has borrowed from the masculine ideal of childhood, from the over-compensation of her feeling of inferiority. If she recoils from a proffer of love or marriage, threatening her as they do with a fresh lowering of her ego-consciousness, she acts symbolically, and all her defensive resources and her predispositions become arrayed against a female destiny and make her seek security where she has always found it, with her father. She utilizes an expedient, behaves in accordance with a senseless fiction, but is nevertheless certain of attaining her goal. The greater her feeling of uncertainty, the more firmly this girl clings to her fiction, endeavors to take it quite literally and since human thinking favors symbolic abstraction the patient with a little effort (and also the analyst) is successful in the longing of neurotics, namely, to find security, to gain a foothold in the symbolic picture of incestuous emotion.

Freud was obliged to see in this purposeful manifestation a reanimation of infantile wishes because according to him the latter are to be looked upon as motive forces. We recognize in this infantile mode of procedure, in the extensive use of safety-devices (Hilfsconstructionen), in which light the neurotic fiction is to be regarded, in the many-sided motor preparedness which reaches into the remote past, in the strong tendency to abstraction and symbolization, the most useful expedient of the neurotic, who strives toward security, toward a maximation of his ego, toward the masculine protest.

If we attach to these critical remarks the question of how the neurotic phenomena come into being, why the patient wills to be a man and constantly seeks to adduce proof thereof, whence he has the stronger necessity for ego-consciousness, why he makes such strong endeavors to gain security, in short, if we inquire into the final reasons for these devices of the neurotic psyche, we may conjecture that which is revealed by every analysis, namely, that at the onset of the development of a neurosis there stands threateningly the feeling of uncertainty and inferiority and demands insistently a guiding, assuring and tranquilizing positing of a goal in order to render life bearable. Among these are especially prominent safety devices and fictions in thought, action and volition.

It is clear that this sort of psyche, directed as it

is with especial force toward a heightening of the
ego, will, aside from specific neurotic symptoms,
make itself conspicuous in society because of its
evident inability to adapt itself. The consciousness of the weak point dominates the neurotic to
such a degree that often without knowing it he
begins to construct with all his might the protecting superstructure. Along with this his sensitiveness becomes more acute, he learns to pay attention to relationships which still escape others,
he exaggerates his cautiousness, begins to anticipate all sorts of disagreeable consequences in
starting out to do something or in experiencing
an injury, he endeavors to hear further and to see
further, belittles himself, becomes insatiable, eco-
nomical, constantly strives to extend the boundaries of his influence and power over space and time
and at the same time loses that peace of mind and
freedom from prejudice which above all guarantee mental health. His mistrust of himself and
others, his envy and maliciousness, become gradually more pronounced, aggressive and cruel
tendencies which are to secure for him supremacy
over his environment, gain the upper hand, or he
endeavors to captivate and conquer others by
means of greater obedience, submission and humility which not infrequently degenerate into
masochistic traits; thus both heightened activity
as well as increased passivity are expedients

ushered in by the fictitious goal of an increased power, of a desire to be above, of the masculine protest.

Thus we have arrived at those psychic phenomena, at the neurotic character, the discussion of which forms the content of this book. None of the neurotic's traits of character are essentially new. He shows no single trait which cannot likewise be demonstrated in the healthy individual, although at times it becomes understandable for the physician as well as the patient only through analysis. It is uninterruptedly "sensitized," thrust forward like an outpost, and represents the sounding of the environment and the future. The knowledge of these psychic dexterities, which protrude far and wide, like sensitive antennæ, first makes possible the understanding of the neurotic's struggle with his fate, of his stimulated aggressive tendency, his unrest and impatience. For these antennæ test all the phenomena of the environment and examine them constantly for their advantages and disadvantages with regard to the assumed goal. They create the keen sense for estimate and comparison, awaken, by means of the attention active in them, fear, hope, doubt, expectations of all sorts and seek to ensure the psyche against surprise and against a lowering of the ego-consciousness. They put forth the most accessible motor dexterities, ever mobile, ever ready to prevent a degradation of the person. The forces of internal and external experience are active in them, they are filled with memory-rests of fear—inspiring as well as consoling experiences, the reminiscences of which they have changed into dexterities. Categorical imperatives of the second rank, they do not serve to bring about their own existence, but in the last analysis cause an elevation of the ego-consciousness and they attempt this by making possible the discovery in the unrest and uncertainty of life, of guiding principles, by facilitating the differentiation between right and wrong, up and down, right and left. The accentuated traits of character are to be found already in the neurotic disposition where they give rise to peculiarities and perversions of conduct. These become still more pronounced when after a more severe attack or after the emergence of a contradiction in the masculine protest, the craving for security (Sicherungstendenz) asserts itself and simultaneously calls forth symptoms as new, effective expedients. They are largely constructed after models and patterns and have for their object the initiation in every new situation of the struggle for the preservation of the ego and victory for it. In their influence lies the reason for the exaggerated affectivity and lowered threshold of stimulation in contrast with normal individuals. It goes without saying that the neurotic character, too, develops out of material already at hand, out of psychic impulses and metamorphosing experiences of the somatic functions.

All these psychic dexterities, standing as they do in close contact with the outside world, become neurotic only when an inner want accentuates the craving for security which in turn more effectively constructs and mobilizes the traits of character only when the fictitious object of life operates more dogmatically and strengthens those secondary guiding principles which are in accord with the traits of character. It is then that the hypostatization of the character sets in, its transformation from a means to a goal leads to an independence of existence and a sort of deification lends to it unchangeability and eternal worth. The neurotic character is thus incapable of adjusting itself to reality because it is always striving toward an impossible ideal. It is a product and instrument of a cautious psyche which strengthens its guiding principle for the purpose of ridding itself of a feeling of inferiority, an attempt which is destined to be wrecked as a consequence of inner contradiction, on the barriers of civilization or on the rights of others. Analogous to the groping gestures, pose in facing the rear, to the bodily attitude in the act of aggression, like mimicry as a form of expression and instrument of motility, so the traits of character, especially the neurotic ones, serve as a psychic means and form of expression for the purpose of entering into an account with life, for the purpose of assuming an attitude, of gaining a fixed point in the vicissitudes of life, for the purpose of reaching that security-giving goal, the feeling of superiority.

Thus we have unmasked the neurotic character as the servant of an imaginary goal and have established its dependence upon a final purpose. It has not sprung up independently out of any sort of biological or constitutional primitive force, but has received direction and motivation from the compensatory superstructure and the schematic guiding principle. Its emergence took place under the pressure of uncertainty, its tendency to personify itself is the doubtful success of the craving for security. This course of the neurotic character has received through the positing of a final purpose its destination which is the masculine main principle and thus every neurotic tendency betrays to us by its direction that it is impregnated with the masculine protest which seeks to make of it an unfailing instrument for the purpose of excluding from experience every permanent degradation.

In the practical part of this book will be shown by means of a series of cases how the "neurotic

scheme" calls forth special psycho-pathological
constellations, namely, through the apperception
of experiences by means of the neurotic character.

INTRODUCTION

Since the inception of the psychoanalytic movement its students have shown a remarkable activity in applying the principles of interpretation originally enunciated by Freud over a wide field of human endeavor, and thus not only have the neurotic and the psychotic come under the critical survey of the analyst, but the whole course of cultural development has been subjected to inquiry along these lines. In addition to this growth in the extent of the movement it has manifested what seems to me to be a very healthy tendency, namely, it has shown an inclination to put forth suggestions as to new methods of approach to the problems, represented here and there by groups of workers who have tended to depart more or less from the original formulations as laid down by Freud. One of the most stimulating and valuable points of view which have been developed in this way is that of Alfred Adler, of Vienna, a translation of whose work on the characteristics of the neurotic character is offered in the following pages.

The distinctive feature of Adler's approach to the problem of the neurotic character traits is that it approaches from the organic rather than from the functional side and in this way, I think, affords a very valuable viewpoint because it tends to bring together the organicist and the

functionalist, who have been too long separated
by the misconception of irreconcilable differences between mind and body. No small part of
the opposition to the whole psychological movement, as represented in psychoanalysis, has come
from the inability of the man who has been
brought up to look at things from the point of
view of the internist to be able to accept many
of the clinical observations which were offered
and which tended to show the development of
clearly organic disorders as a result of a dis-
turbance in the psyche. Adler's approach to the
psychoanalytic problems is admirably calculated
to break down such prejudices.

In this book, however, the working out of the
significance of the various neurotic character
traits has been by ringing the changes on the
basic formulation of what Adler calls the masculine protest. It is as if the neurotic said to
himself, " I wish to be a complete man." This
protest arises on the basis of a feeling of inferiority and an effort upon the part of the
neurotic to correct this feeling, which he does
by so ordering his life, so regulating his every
act that he may find that security of which the
feeling of inferiority has robbed him. This is the
fictitious goal of the neurotic and the fundamental and ultimate cause of his symptoms when
he is no longer able to succeed, when failure
threatens in his efforts to deal with reality.

For Adler the neurosis or the psychosis is
comparable to the work of art, but has been
built up in response to a fictitious goal which

collects and unites into a group those psychic elements of which it can make use, collecting only those which promise results in the effort at the attainment of security. The attempt to attain to the maximation of his ego fails because directed along a false path. The neurosis or psychosis is therefore a constructive creation, a compensation product, which, however, fails because of its false direction.

All this is very psychological and does not bear out what I have said about it to the effect that Adler's approach is from the organic side. This particular book, however, stresses the psychological formula. In his earlier work on organ inferiority [1] the organic basis of this psychological formulation is founded. The feeling of inferiority, which underlies the masculine protest, has its raison d'être in an inferior organ.

In this work he has gone to considerable extent in working over the psychological characteristics of persons who have had demonstrably inferior organs, either clinically evident or showing up at autopsy. From this work he believes he has been able to show that the predominant traits of character are the result of an effort on the part of the individual to overcome a feeling of inferiority resulting from an inferior organ. Many examples might be given, and in fact they come within the ken of every one, which demonstrate the validity of this point of view. A classical example is that of Demosthenes, a stam-

[1] Translation in preparation, as Number 24 of the Nervous and Mental Disease Monograph Series.

merer, who became the greatest orator of Greece. Adler believes that defects of this sort nucleate, so to say, the feeling of inferiority and force the individual to make supreme efforts to overcome his particular defect and in this way, as a result of these efforts, the inferior organ, by the development of a highly differentiated nervous superstructure, may actually become supernormal, a result which we are familiar with, for example, in the remarkable facility with which blind people gain information through their supersensitized touch organs. In other words, to use the language of current psychoanalysis, the organ inferiority is the basic factor of what the Freudians refer to as the conflict.

These two works of Adler's, therefore, give the organic basis and the psychological elaboration of his opinions. The neurotic constitution founds in an inferior organ, the inferior organ produces a feeling of inferiority, the feeling of inferiority—the masculine protest—becomes the fictitious goal of the neurotic, whose symptoms result from an effort to mould reality along this false pathway.

To those who follow Adler through the various ramifications of his hypothesis, who read sympathetically his numerous case reports which he offers to substantiate his views, there can be no doubt but that the angle from which he looks at the problem of the neuroses and the psychoses lets us see new aspects of these phenomena which are exceedingly helpful to us in our effort to grasp their meanings. It will also be perfectly evident that the helpfulness of the Adler theories is in the orientation which the physician gets towards the problem presented by the patient, whether he approach it from the point of view of the internist or of the psychologist. Adler's theories are admirably calculated to help the internist to grasp the possibilities of organ inferiority as they may affect the psyche and to help the psychoanalyst to grasp the origin and meanings of the neurosis as he sees it at the psychological level and perhaps to see more clearly upon what his limitations are based. In any event the two groups of physicians, heretofore separated all too far, both in theory and practice, may find in Adler's views a common ground upon which to meet.

WILLIAM A. WHITE.

SAINT ELIZABETH'S HOSPITAL,
    WASHINGTON, D. C.
October 23, 1916.

CONTENTS

CONTENTS

THE NEUROTIC CONSTITUTION

THE
NEUROTIC CONSTITUTION

CHAPTER I

THE ORIGIN AND DEVELOPMENT OF THE FEELING OF INFERIORITY AND THE CONSEQUENCES THEREOF

THE facts established through my study of somatic inferiority (*vide* Studie, *l.c.*) concerned themselves with the causes, the behavior, the manifestations and altered mode of activity of inferiorily developed organs and has led me to assume the idea of "compensation through the central nervous system" with which were linked certain discussions of the subject of psychogenesis.

There came to light a remarkable relationship between somatic inferiority and psychic overcompensation, so that I gained a fundamental viewpoint, namely, that the realization of somatic inferiority by the individual becomes for him a permanent impelling force for the development of his psyche.

Physiologically there results from this a reënforcement of the nerve tracts, both quantitatively and qualitatively, whereby a concomitant original inferiority of these tracts is enabled to reveal in a composite picture its tectonic and functional peculiarities.

The psychic phase of this compensation and overcompensation can only be disclosed by means of psychologic investigation and analysis.

As I have given a detailed description of organ-inferiority as the etiology of the neuroses in my former contributions, especially in the "Studie," in the "Aggressionstrieb," in "Psychischen Her-maphroditismus," in the "Neurotischen Disposi-tion" and in the "Psychischen Behandlung der Trigeminusneuralgie," I may in the present de-scription confine myself to those points which promise a further elucidation of the relationship between somatic-inferiority and psychic compen-sation and which are of importance in the study of the neurotic character.

Summarizing, I lay stress on the fact that organ-inferiority, as described by me, includes the incompleteness in such organs, the frequently demonstrable arrests of development or func-tional maturity, the functional failure in the post-fetal period and the fetal character of organs and systems of organs; on the other hand the accen-tuation of their developmental tendency in the presence of compensatory and coördinating forces and the frequent bringing about of increased functional activity. One may easily detect in every instance from observation of the child and from the anamneses of the adult that the possession of definitely inferior organs is reflected upon the psyche—and in such a way as to lower the self-esteem, to raise the child's psychological uncertainty; but it is just out of this lowered self-esteem that there arises the struggle for self-assertion which assumes forms much more intense than one would expect. As the compensated inferior organ gains in the scope of activity both qualitatively and quantitatively and acquires protective means from itself as well as from the entire organism, the predisposed child in his sense of inferiority selects out of his psychic resources expedients for the raising of his own value which are frequently striking in nature and among which may be noted as occupying the most prominent places those of a neurotic and psychotic character.

Ideas concerning innate inferiority, predisposition, and constitutional weakness may be found even in the very beginnings of scientific medicine. In leaving out of discussion here many noteworthy contributions, although they frequently contained fundamental viewpoints, we do so solely because the relationship between organic and psychic disease states, albeit dwelt upon, was

never explained. In this class belong all viewpoints of pathology which are founded upon a
general assumption of degeneracy. Stiller's
theory of the asthenic habitus goes considerably
further and almost attempts to establish etiologi-
cal relationships. Anton's compensation theory
confines itself all too closely to correlation systems
within the central nervous system; nevertheless,
he, as well as his talented pupil, Otto Gross, have
made noteworthy attempts to bring about on this
basis a clearer understanding of certain psychotic
states. Bouchard's bradytrophy, the exudative
diathesis described by Ponflick, Escherich,
Czerny, Moro and Strümpel, and interpreted by
them as a disease-producing diathesis, Comby's
infantile arthritism, Kreibich's angio-neurotic
diathesis, Heubner's lymphatism, Poltauf's status
thymico-lymphaticus, Escherich's spasmophilia
and Hess-Eppinger's vagotonia are successful
attempts of recent decades to describe disease
states associated with congenital inferiority.

All of them refer to heredity and infantile
characteristics. But, although the vague and in-
constant limits of the predispositions in question
are emphasized by the authors themselves, the
impression is not to be ignored that certain conspicuous types have been isolated which in the
course of time will be brought within one large
group, namely, that of the minus-variants.   Of

extreme importance for the understanding of congenital inferiority and predisposition to disease are the researches into the glands of internal secretion in which morphologic as well as functional deviations have been discovered, e.g., the thyroids, the parathyroids, the sex glands, the chromaffin system and the hypophysis. Considered from the standpoint of their organ-inferiorities the orientation of the composite picture becomes easier and the relationship to compensation and correlation in the economy of the entire body becomes clearer. Among the remaining investigators who took as the basis for their views not a primum-movens, but a combined influence of various organ-inferiorities and mutual interaction of the same, Martius, above all, must be mentioned. In my contribution on "The Inferiority of Organs" (1907), the idea of the coördination of the coexisting inferiorities likewise appears prominently. The fact is not to be lightly evaluated that the simultaneously existing organ-inferiorities stand in relation to one another as if united by a secret bond.

Bartel likewise has extended his theories concerning the status thymico-lymphaticus, which represents a considerable advance in science, to such limits as to invade the boundaries of the systems of other authors. Kyrle too, supporting himself by the newly discovered pathological findings, reached quite independently conclusions identical with mine, namely, that the coördination of the inferiority of the sexual apparatus with other organ-inferiorities, though frequently only slightly developed, is nevertheless so often found to exist that I must maintain that there exist no organ-inferiorities without an accompanying defect in the sexual apparatus.

Because of some future considerations I must also mention certain of the views of Freud who assumes a sexual constitution as the basis of the neuroses and psychoses, under which term he understands a qualitatively and quanitatively varying arrangement of partial sex impulses. This assumption simply corresponds to a postulate advanced by him for his other views. The development of perverse inclinations and their unsuccessful repression into the unconscious furnishes, according to him, the picture of the neurosis, and in itself forms the primary cause for the neurotic psyche. We shall see from our considerations that perversion so far as it reaches development in the neurosis and psychosis is not dependent upon a connate impulse, but that it arises from the striving towards a fictitious goal in connection with which the repression takes place as a by-product under the pressure of the self-consciousness.

That which, however, is to be taken cognizance

of biologically in an originally abnormal sexual conduct, namely, the greater or lesser sensitiveness, the heightened or lowered reflex activity, the functional valency as well as the compensatory psychic superstructure indicates directly as I have shown in my "Studie" a congenital defect of the sexual organ.

Concerning the nature of the predisposition to disease dependent upon organ-inferiority there exists a unanimity of opinion. The standpoint assumed by me ("Studie," *l.c.*) emphasizes more strongly than does that of other authors, the assurance of an adjustment through compensation. With the release from the maternal organism there begins for these inferior organs or systems of organs the struggle with the outside world, which must of necessity ensue and which is initiated with greater vehemence than in the more normally developed apparatus. This struggle is accompanied by greater mortality and morbidity rates. This fetal character, however, at the same time furnishes the increased possibility for compensation and over-compensation, increases the adaptability to ordinary and extraordinary resistances and assures the attainment of new and higher forms, new and higher accomplishments.

Thus the inferior organs furnish the inexhaustible material by means of which the organism continuously seeks to reach a better accord with the altered conditions of life through adaptation, repudiation, and improvement. Its hypervalency is deeply rooted in the compulsion of a constant training, in the variability and greater tendency to growth, frequently associated with inferior organs, and in the more facile evolution of the appertaining nervous and psychic complexes, on account of the introspection and concentration bestowed on them. The evils of constitutional inferiority manifest themselves in the most varied diseases and predispositions to disease.

At times various somatic or mental disabilities develop, at other times an over-irritability of the nerve tracts, then again clumsiness of manner, ungainliness, precocity. A host of childhood defects coöperate with the predisposition to disease and form a close union, as I have shown, with the organic or functional inferiority. Strabismus, anomalies of refraction of the visual apparatus or photophobia with its train of symptoms, deafmutism, stuttering and other defects of speech, difficulty of hearing, the organic and psychic defects which go with adenoid vegetations, the complete aprosexia, the frequent affections of the sensory organs, of the respiratory and digestive tracts, striking ugliness and deformities, peripheral stigmata of degeneration and nævi which may indicate more profound organ-inferiorities

(Alder, Schmidt). Hydrocephalus, rickets, anomalies of stature as scoliosis, round shoulders, genu varus or valgus, pes varus or valgus, a protracted incontinence of feces and urine, malformations of the genitals, results of small arteries (Virchow) and the numerous consequences of defects of the internal secretory glands as described by Wagner v. Yauregg, Frankl v. Hochwert, Chvostek, Bartel, Escherich, Pineles and others, all of which reveal in their great abundance, in the variety of their combinations, the large sphere of disease manifestations as disclosed to the physician through an understanding of organ-inferiority. It was especially pediatrists and pathologists who first noted these relationships. But the concept of degeneracy has likewise become of increasing importance to neurology and psychiatry. The line of advance stretches all the way from Morel's theory of the stigmata of degeneration to the consideration of nervous diseases from the standpoint of an inferior constitution. We need only consider the statistical study of Thiemich-Birks and Potpeschnigg's contributions (cited by Gött) concerning the fate of children who were treated in the first and second years of their lives for tetanoid convulsions. Of these children only a small number became entirely well. In most instances there were found later definite signs of somatic and psychic inferiority, psychopathic and neuropathic characteristics. As such, these authors mention infantilism, squints, difficulty of hearing, speech defects, feeble-mindedness, disturbances of sleep, pavor nocturnus, somnambulism, enuresis, exaggerated reflexes, tics, paroxysms of rage, truancy, timidity, pathological lying and habitual fugues.

Gött as well as other authors reached the conclusion that in spasmophilic children there exists a predisposition to severe neurotic and psychopathic states. Czerny and others maintain that a similar relationship may be found in children suffering from gastro-intestinal disorders.

Bartel was able to discover among suicides a considerable preponderance of the status thymico-lymphaticus, especially a hypoplasia of the sexual organs. The existence of somatic inferiority among juvenile suicides was shown by me, Netslitzky and others. Frankl v. Hochwert described states of excitement, irritability and hallucinatory confusion, in tetany. French writers (cited from Pfaundler) ascribe to the torpid habitus of children, moroseness, indolence, sleepiness, distractibility, stupidity and phlegmatism, to the erotistic type, restlessness, liveliness, irritability, precocity, moodiness, affectivity, unsociability, peculiarity of disposition and one-sided development. Pfaundler emphasizes the harassing, tormenting and painful influences to which

defective children are subject as a result of skin
eruptions, colic, disturbances of sleep and functional anomalies. Czerny, who called attention
to the relationship between intestinal disturbances of children and neuroses, emphasizes especially the importance of psychotherapy in children who became neurotic in the course of constitutional diseases. Only recently Hamburger has
thrown light upon the nature of the ambitions in
neurotic children, while Stransky showed the relation between myopathy and psychic manifestations.

These brief references give us an insight into
the attempts of the present day scientific trends
to emphasize and maintain the relation between
psychic anomalies in childhood and constitutional
inferiority. The first comprehensive fundamental views concerning this relation were published by me in the "Studie," wherein I showed
how the inferior organ constantly endeavors to
make a very special demand upon the interest and
attention. I was able to prove in this and other
contributions to what extent inferiority of an
organ constantly shows its influence on the psyche
in action, in thought, in dreams, in the choice of a
vocation and in artistic inclinations and capabilities.[1]

[1] See also Adler, "The Theory of Organ-inferiority and Its
Significance for Philosophy and Psychology." Address in the

The existence of an inferior organ demands a kind of training on the part of the appertaining nerve tracts and on the part of the psychic super-structure which would render the latter active in a compensatory manner when a possibility for compensation exists.   In such an event, however, we must likewise find a reënforcement in the psychic superstructure of certain allied points of contact which the inferior organ has with the outside world.

To the originally inferior organ of vision corresponds a reënforced visual psyche; a defective digestive apparatus will be accompanied by a greater psychic capability in all nutritional directions, as gourmondism, acquisitiveness, and where it concerns money equivalents, stinginess and greed, will be manifested to an extraordinary degree.

The ability of the compensating nervous system will manifest itself through qualified reflexes (Adler) and conditioned reflexes (Bickel) by means of sensitive reactions and exaggerated sensitiveness.   The compensating psychic super-structure will bring about an accentuated manifestation of the psychic phenomena of presentiments and forethoughts and their effective factors such as memory, intuition, introspection,

Philosophic Society of the Vienna University, 1908, and J. Reich, "Art and the Eye," Oesterreichische Rundschau, 1908.

analysis, attention, hypersensitiveness, in brief, of all the fortifying psychic forces. To these reassuring forces belong also the fixation and accentuation of those traits which form useful guiding principles in the chaos of life, thus diminishing the feeling of uncertainty.

The neurotic individual is derived from this sphere of uncertainty and in his childhood is under the pressure of his constitutional inferiority. In most cases this may be easily detected. In other cases the patient behaves as if he were inferior. In all cases, however, his striving and thinking are built upon the foundation of the feeling of inferiority. This feeling must always be understood in a relative sense, as the outgrowth of the individual's relation to his environment or to his strivings. He has constantly been drawing comparisons between himself and others, at first with his father, as the strongest in the family, sometimes with his mother, his brothers and sisters, later with every person with whom he comes into contact. Upon closer analysis, one finds that every child, especially the one less favored by nature, has made a careful estimate of his own value. The constitutionally inferior child, the unattractive child, the child too strictly reared, the pampered child, all of whom we may align as being predisposed to the development of a neurosis, seek more diligently than does the normal child to avoid the evils of their existence. They soon long to banish into a distant future the fate which confronts them. In order to bring this about, he, the defective child, requires an expedient which enables him to keep before his eyes a fixed picture in the vicissitudes of life and the uncertainty of his existence. He turns to the construction of this expedient. He sums up in his self-estimation all evils, considers himself incompetent, inferior, degraded, insecure. And in order to find a guiding principle he takes as a second fixed point his father or mother who endowed him with all the attributes of life.

And in adjusting this guiding principle to his thinking and acting, in his endeavors to raise himself to the level of his (all-powerful) father, even to the point of surpassing the latter, he has quite removed himself with one mighty bound from reality and is suspended in the meshes of a fiction.

Similar observations may also be made in a lesser degree among normal children. They too desire to be great, to be strong, to rule as the father, and are guided by this objective. Their conduct, their psychical and physical attitude is constantly directed towards this goal, so that one may almost detect a true imitation, an identical psychic gesture.

Example becomes the guide to the "masculine"

goal, so long as the masculinity is not doubted. Should the idea of "the masculine goal" become unacceptable to girls, then there takes place a change of form of this "masculine" guiding principle. One can scarcely evaluate this phenomenon in a more correct way than by assuming that the necessary denial of the gratification of certain organic functions forces the child from the first hour of his extrauterine life into assuming a combative attitude towards his environment. From this result tensions and accentuations of certain organically acquired abilities—*c'est la guerre!*— as I have described them in my "Studie" and the "Aggressionstrieb." [2]

In the temporary denials and discomforts which the first years of childhood bring with them, one must seek the impulse for the development of a host of common traits of character. Above all the child learns, in his weakness and helplessness, in his anxiety and manifold shortcomings to value an expedient which assures him of the help and support of his relatives and guarantees their concern. In his negativistic behavior, in his obstinacy and refractoriness, he often finds a gratification of his consciousness of his own powers, thus ridding himself of the painful realization of his inferiority. Both main-

[2] Adler, "Der Aggressionstrieb im Leben und in der Neurose," l. c.

springs of the child's behavior, obstinacy and obedience (Adler, "Trotz and Gehorsam") guarantee to him an accentuation of his feeling of ego-consciousness and assist him in groping his way towards the masculine goal or, as we wished to adduce before, towards the equivalent of this. The awakening self-consciousness is always being suppressed in constitutionally inferior children, their self-esteem is lowered because their capacity for gratification is much more limited.

Let us consider the numerous restrictions, the courses of treatment and the sufferings of children ill with gastro-intestinal derangements; the effeminacy and fastidiousness seen in the anæmic, weakly children suffering from respiratory disorders; the itching and tortures of those afflicted with prurigo and other exanthemata; the many degrading defects of childhood; the fear of contamination on the part of the parents of such children which often leads, as do the frequent difficulties in their bringing up—in their school progress as well as the stubbornness of these children—to an isolation and misunderstanding on the part of their comrades and within the family circle.   In the same manner the self-consciousness is injured by rachitic clumsiness, congenital obesity and the lesser grades of mental backwardness.   The child usually explains his difficulty by the assumption of a neglect, a slight by the parents, especially as it occurs in later children or in the youngest, occasionally even in the first born. This hostile aggression, reënforced and accentuated in constitutionally inferior children, becomes confluent with his effort to become as great and strong as the strongest and thrusts forward activities which lie at the bottom of the infantile ambition. All later trains of thought and activities of the neurotic are constructed similarly with his childhood wish phantasy. The "recurrence of the identical" (Nietzsche) is nowhere so well illustrated as in the neurotic. His feeling of inferiority in the presence of men and things, his uncertainty in the world force him to an accentuation of his guiding principles. To these he clings throughout life in order to orient himself in existence by means of his beliefs and superstitions, in order to overcome his feeling of inferiority, in order to rescue his sense of ego-consciousness, in order to possess a subterfuge to avoid a much-dreaded degradation. Never has he succeeded so well in this as during his childhood. His guiding fiction which makes him behave as if he surpassed all others may therefore also bring about a form of conduct identical with that of the child.

In such manner then the infantile gratifications become criteria and thus strengthen the guiding principle. It would be amiss to assume that only the neurotic exhibits such "guiding principles." The healthy individual would also have to do without orientation in the world if he did not arrange the cosmic picture and his experience according to some imaginary fiction. In hours of uncertainty these fictions come to the fore more distinctly and become the imperative influences dominating beliefs, ideals and free will; moreover they also act secretly in the unconscious like all other psychic mechanisms whose verbal image they represent in conscious thought. Logically considered they are to be regarded as abstractions, as simplifications, which have for their object the solution of life's difficulties in a manner analogous to that required for the simplest experiences. The original type of these simplest experiences, the meshwork of apperceptive memory, we found in studying the child's efforts to solve his difficulties. In dreams this form of apperception is still more obvious; we shall consider this subject later.

The neurotic carries his feeling of inferiority constantly with him. Hence his method of thinking by analogy is more strongly and clearly developed.

His "misoneism" (Lombroso), his fear of the new, of decisions and tests, which is usually present, originates from the lack of analogy for these new conditions. He has chained himself so strongly to guiding principles, taken them so literally and sought to realize them only, that unconsciously he has become incapable of proceeding freely and without prejudice to the solution of real problems. Even the necessary limitations imposed by reality, where matters clash for want of room, do not impel him to reject his fiction because he is forced to suspend it, but only to alter it. Still more consequentially the psychotic patient strives to bring about a realization of his fiction. The neurotic in real life flounders in his self-created guiding principle and thus arrives at a splitting of the personality in seeking to do justice to both the real and the imaginary requirements. The form and content of the neurotic "guiding principle" originate from the impressions of the child who feels himself neglected. These impressions, which of necessity develop out of an original sense of inferiority, call forth an aggressive attitude in life, the object of which is the overcoming of the uncertainty. In this attitude of aggression all those efforts of the child which tend toward an elevation of his feeling of ego-consciousness find their place, successful efforts which prompt a repetition, unsuccessful ones which serve as mementoes for those goal-preparing tendencies developed out of a conspicuous organic disease and which express themselves in a mass of psychic predispositions, as well as those observed in others. All the phenomena of the neuroses originate from these predisposing means which tend toward the attainment of the final object, masculinity. They are mental predispositions always ready to initiate the struggle for ego-consciousness, they obey the command of the guiding principle which seeks to realize itself through the channels of reactions lying ready at hand in childhood. In the developed neuroses the fiction stimulates all these predispositions whereupon they comport themselves as independent final purposes. Anxiety, which formerly sought to furnish assurance against being alone, against underestimation, against the feeling of insignificance, is hypostasized; the compulsion, originally in the sense of the fiction to preserve a manly behavior, becomes independent; in fainting, in paralysis, in the hysterical pains and functional disturbances, the pseudo-masochistic method of the patient is symbolically represented, in which he seeks to attract attention or to avoid a decision which is feared. The important rôle played by the neurotic uncertainty, as I have recognized and described it, leads to that sort of strengthening of the predisposition and its consequences which makes the originally unimportant phenomena of a functional nature assume the most astonishing exaggeration as soon as the inner exigency demands it.

The gaze of the neurotic, on account of this feeling of uncertainty, is directed far into the future. All present existence is to him only a preparation. Moreover this circumstance is largely responsible for encouraging his dreaming proclivities and estranging him from the world of reality. As with religious persons his kingdom is not of this world and like them he cannot free himself from his self-created deity, the exaltation of his ego-consciousness. A host of general traits of character of necessity develop in an individual thus turned away from reality. First of all must be mentioned the deep reverence in which are held the expedients which subserve the fiction. An individual of this type will as a rule manifest a carefully adjusted mode of behavior, exactness and pedantry, first of all, in order not to increase the great difficulties of life and secondly and principally, in order to distinguish himself from others in dress, in work, in morals, and thus acquire for himself a feeling of superiority. This exaggerated trait of character usually serves also to bring him face to face with the enemy, to furnish the opportunity for a maturing of such situations as will bring him into conflict with his environment so that he finds occasion for giving vent to reproaches. At the same time these constant reproaches serve to keep alive his feeling, his attention, to the fact that people are neglecting him, that they are not taking him into account.   This trait may be found even in the childhood of certain neurotics where it serves the purpose of putting some one at their service, say the mother, who must take care of their clothes every evening for a considerable length of time in a definitely prescribed manner.   In a similarly remarkable manner, anxiety and timidity gain expression and I must adhere to the opinion, in spite of all other attempts at explanation, that the psychic phenomena of anxiety originate from an hallucinatory excitation of a predisposition which in childhood developed automatically from small beginnings as soon as a bodily injury was threatened, and which in later life, especially in the neuroses, is conditioned by the final goal, namely, to escape a lowering of ego-consciousness and to make oneself of service to others.   It is easy to understand how all wish-phantasies may attain an enormous degree, just as attainment seldom brings with it satisfaction.   One may assume without fear of contradiction that a neurotic "wishes to have everything."   This desire coincides with his "guiding fiction" to become potent. If he draws back in horror before undertakings which promise advantage, as he usually does before crimes and immoral acts, it is because he entertains fears for the safety of his ego-consciousness.   For this reason he recoils in horror from lying, but in order to proceed with certainty and in order to preserve steadfastness he may harbor the thought that he is capable of great evils and crimes. That this obstinate pursuit of the fiction implies a social injury is obvious.

The egoism of neurotics, their envy, their greed, frequently unconscious, their tendency to undervalue men and things, originate in their feeling of uncertainty and serve the purpose of assuring them, of guiding them and of spurring them on. As they are enveloped in phantasy and live in the future their preoccupation is not to be wondered at. The variability of temper depends on the play of the phantasy which at one time awakens painful memories, at another fills with the enthusiasm of an expected triumph, analogous to the vacillations and doubts of the neurotic. In the same way special traits of character which are not foreign to the normal psyche appear to be directed by the hypnotizing goal and strengthened in this direction. Sexual precocity and falling in love are forms of expression for the heightened tendency to captivate. Masturbation, impotence and perverse excitements lie in the direction of the guiding line of fear of a partner and fear of separation, along with which sadism represents the desire to play the "wild man" in order to overcome the feeling of inferiority. As the driving force and goal of the neurosis developing out of a constitutional inferiority, we have up to this point regarded the accentuation of ego-consciousness which constantly strives for expression with especial force. In doing so we have not ignored the fact that this is only a mode of expression of a striving and yearning whose beginnings are deeply rooted in human nature. The form of expression itself and the accentuation of this guiding thought, which may also be expressed by Nietzsche's "will to power," teaches us that there is an especial compensatory force at play, whose object it is to put an end to the inner uncertainty. By means of an unyielding formula, which usually presses to the surface of consciousness, the neurotic seeks to obtain the fulcrum whereby to lift the world off of its hinges. It matters but little how much of this driving force becomes consciously known to the neurotic. The mechanism itself he never understands, neither is he able to explain and break down unaided his mode of apperception by means of analogy and the conduct resulting therefrom. This can only succeed by means of an analytic process which permits us to divine and understand his infantile analogy by means of abstraction, reduction and simplification. In this way one finds regularly apparent that the neurotic always apperceives after the analogy of a contrast, indeed, that usually he only recognizes and gives value to relations of contrast. This primitive mode of orientation in life which corresponds to the antithesis as set forth in the categories of Aristotle and to opposites in the Pythagorean table originates also in the feeling of uncertainty and illustrates a simple device of logic. What I have described as polar, hermaphroditic opposites, Lombroso as bipolar, Bleuler as ambivalent, leads to this same method of apperception which works according to the principal of opposites. One should not fall into the common error of regarding this as an essence of things, but must recognize in it the primitive method of procedure which measures a thing, a force, or an event, by an opposite which is fitted to it.

The further the analysis proceeds the more distinct appears one of these opposites, the original form of which we have established as the feeling of inferiority and the maximation of the ego-consciousness. This only agrees with the primitive efforts of the child to orient himself in the world and to obtain certainty when tangible antitheses are encountered. Among these I have regularly found the following: (1). Above—beneath, (2). Masculine—feminine. One furthermore always finds an arrangement of memories, feelings and actions according to this type of antitheses in the sense the patient takes them (not always in the generally accepted sense), i.e., inferior—beneath, feminine; powerful—above, masculine. This grouping is important for it renders possible, because it can be conserved or falsified at will, the distortion of the cosmic picture, whereby the neurotic can always hold fast to his standpoint, namely, that of a neglected person, by rearrangement, by accentuation or by arbitrary changes. It lies in the nature of things that in this process his constitutional inferiority comes to his assistance as well as his constantly increasing aggressive environment which is continually set into activity by the neurotic conduct of the patient.

At times the neurotic is not fully conscious of his supposed or real defeat. It is then always found that it is his pride which prevents him from recognizing it. Nevertheless he acts as if he had appreciated the new degradation and the riddle of a nervous attack is often only solved when this fact is understood. The revelation of such repressed feelings is not of much therapeutic value, at least, it can only be of value when by means of it the connection with the infantile mechanism which is responsible for the predisposition to the attack becomes apparent to the patient. At times there results even a seeming relapse which may be explained by the fact that the patient directs his predispositions against the physician because the latter has injured his feelings of personal worth.

There still remains to be answered one important question. On what does the patient base his feeling of inferiority? Inasmuch as the patient is only able to detect the possibility of relationship between disease predispositions and those organ-inferiorities which force themselves upon his attention he is constantly in the path of conjecture. He will for example not seek the reason for his inferiorities in the disturbances of the secretions of the glands, but will blame in a general way his weakness, his stunted growth, his sham education, the small size or anomalies of his genitals, lack of complete virility, his effeminacy, the feminine traits of a physical or psychic nature, his parents, his heredity; at times only lack of love, bad training, deprivation in childhood, etc. And what about his neurosis, the neurosis in the sense we understand it? We shall find that the accentuation of his predispositions on an analogic, childish basis, that his symbolized thoughts, his preparations for feelings, and results used by him as means of expression will spring into action as soon as the patient fears or experiences a set-back. Being from a certain situation, so to speak, inoculated with the feelings of inferiority, he exhibits an anaphylactic reaction against depreciation of his ego-consciousness and finds in irresolution, in vacillation, in doubt and in skepticism, as well as in the breaking out of a neurosis or a psychosis, a refuge and security against the greatest evil that could befall him, namely, the conjuring up of a distinct realization of his inferiority. In line with this the typical causes of the onset of a neurosis and psychosis are easy to divine and to prove:

1. The desire for knowledge of sex differences, the uncertainty concerning his own sexual rôle, may be looked upon as causes of the arousing of the feeling of inferiority. Likewise the realization and grouping of traits believed to be feminine, the vacillating, doubting, hermaphrodistic apperception and hermaphrodistic predisposition. Predisposition to and psychic gestures of the feminine rôle always entail greater passivity, anxious anticipation, etc., but call forth the masculine protest, stronger emotivity. (Heymanns)

2. Onset of menstruation.
3. Epoch of menstrual activity.
4. Epoch of sexual activity.
5. The stage of fitness for marriage.
6. Pregnancy.
7. Puerperium.
8. Climacteric, reduction of potency.
9. Examinations, choice of profession.
10. Danger of death.

All these epochs call forth heightening of or changes in the preparatory attitude toward life. The bond common to them all which holds them together is the expectation of new events which imply for the neurotic new struggles, new dangers of a set-back. He proceeds therefore immediately to intensive protective measures, the most extreme of which is suicide. Outbreaks of neuroses and psychoses represent accentuations of his neurotic preparedness, predispositions in which are always found prominent traits of character, calculated to guarantee this sort of security, such as exaggeration of hypersensitiveness, greater carefulness, irritability, pedantry, obstinacy, stinginess, discontent, impatience, and many others. As these traits are easily demonstrable, they are especially suitable for determining the existence of a psychogenic disorder.

We arrived at the conclusion in the foregoing that it is the feeling of uncertainty which forces the neurotic to a stronger attachment to fictions, guiding principles, ideals, dogmas. These guiding principles float before the normal person also. But to him they are a figure of speech, a device for distinguishing above from below, left from right, right from wrong, and he is not so involved in prejudice that when called upon to make a decision he cannot free himself from the abstract and reckon with reality. Just as little do the phenomena of life resolve themselves for him into strict antitheses, but on the contrary he is striving constantly to keep his thoughts and actions detached from this unreal principle and to bring them into harmony with reality. That he uses artifices at all as a means to an end arises from the usefulness of the fiction in casting up the accounts of life. The neurotic, however, like the child devoid of contact with life and like the primitive understanding of early man catches at the straw of his fiction, hypostasizes it, arbitrarily ascribes to it a real value and seeks to realize it in the world. For this the fiction is unfitted, still more unfitted when, as in the psychoses, it is elevated to a dogma or anthropomorphosed. The symbol as a "modus dicendi" dominates our speech and thought. The neurotic takes it literally and in the psychosis the realization is attempted. In my contributions to the theory of the neuroses this point is constantly emphasized and maintained. A fortunate circumstance made me acquainted with Vaihinger's ingenious "Philosophy of the 'As If'" (Berlin, 1911), a work in which I found the trains of thought suggested to me by the neurosis set forth as valid for general scientific thought.

After we have established that the fictitious guiding goal of the neurotic consists of an unlimited heightening of the ego-consciousness which deteriorates into the "will to seem" (Nietzsche) we may proceed to a consideration of the abstract conception of these problems of life. Inasmuch as in seeking the sex differentiation the rôle of the male is given a decided preference, the formal changes agreeing with the antithesis, man-woman, begin at an early period and for the neurotic arises the formula " I must act as though I were a complete man (or would become one)." The feeling of inferiority and its consequences become identified with the feeling of effeminacy, the compensatory pressure in the psychic super-structure impels toward obtaining a guarantee that the manly rôle will be preserved and the meaning of the neurosis assumes the form of the antithetical, fundamental thought, "I am a woman and will be a man."

This guiding final purpose supplies the psychic gestures and predispositions necessary for this thought, but is expressed likewise in the attitudes of the body and in mimicry. And with these prepared gestures, of which the neurotic traits of character are to be considered a heralding, the neurotic confronts persons and life, anxiously and with strained attention asking if he will prove himself a man. Sham combats play a great rôle; they are begun so that the neurotic may exercise himself, that he may gain experience from other or similar conditions, so that he may become more cautious, and in order to obtain proof from example that he dare not venture upon the main battle. How much in this he re-

arranges, exaggerates, depreciates, which is possible to him from a certain arbitrariness (Meyer-
hoff), how he falsely classifies and how he seeks
to put his fiction on firm foundation, demand a
separate consideration, such as I have tentatively
furnished in the preliminary work for this book.
That in this masculine protest, however, there
lies for the neurotic the more fundamentally compensating "will to power" which may change the
value of feelings and even transform pleasure
into pain is proved by the frequent cases where
the direct effort to act like a man meets with obstacles and avails itself of a circuitous route, in
which event the rôle of the woman is overvalued,
passive traits are strengthened, masochistic, and
in men, passive homosexual traits emerge, by
means of which the patient hopes to gain power
over men and women: in short, the masculine
protest makes use of the feminine rôle in order to
attain its purpose.

That this device is likewise dictated by the
"will to power" is proved by the further neurotic
traits which strive for mastery and superiority in
the most extreme form. This apperception,
however, brings the sexual jargon into the neurosis which must be regarded as symbolic and requires interpretation.

Side by side with or dominating it is found in
neurotics the method of apperception which ar-

ranges perception according to the spatial antithesis, above-beneath. Also, for this primitive
attempt at orientation, which the neurotic emphasizes very strongly, one finds analogies in primitive people. However, while it is easy to understand that the masculine principle is identified
with perfection, we are forced to guesses in regard to the valuation of "above" as the equal of
the principle. A certain probability seems to
give color to the opinion that the value and significance of the upper part of the body in comparison with the feet furnishes the explanation.
Still more important it seems to me that the valuation of the word above and its covaluation with
perfection originates in the longing of man to
lift himself, to fly, to do that which is impossible
for man. The universal flying dreams and the
efforts of man in the same direction seem to confirm this opinion. That in the congressus sex-
ualis the "above" is confluent with the masculine
principle does not seem without significance.

The reënforcement of the fiction in the neurosis causes a concentration of the attention on
those points of view regarded by the neurotic as
important. Therefrom results the narrowing of
the field of vision and the psychic preparation as
motor and psychic predispositions. Simultaneously, the more accentuated neurotic character
comes into force, which maintains the assurance

of the fiction, comes in touch with inimical forces and, spreading itself out far over the boundaries of personality, into the realms of space and time, furnishes, in the form of a secondary guiding line, an impetus to the will to power. The neurotic attack, finally, like the strife for power, has for its purpose the protection of the ego-consciousness from degradation.

Therefore from constitutional inferiority there arises a feeling of inferiority which demands a compensation in the sense of a maximation of the ego-consciousness. From this circumstance the fiction which serves as a final purpose acquires an astonishing influence and draws all the psychic forces in its direction. Itself an outgrowth of the striving for security, it organizes psychic preparatory measures for the purpose of guaranteeing security, among which the neurotic character as well as the functional neurosis are noticeable as prominent devices.

The guiding fiction has a simple, infantile scheme, and influences the apperception and the mechanism of memory.

CHAPTER II

OUR examination of the facts has led us to understand how out of the absolute inferiority of the child (especially the one constitutionally burdened), there is evolved a kind of self estimation which calls forth a feeling of inferiority.

Analogously to the δός ποῦ στῶ the child seeks to gain a standpoint which will enable him to get a perspective in the problems of life. From this point of departure, which is taken as a fixed pole in the flux of phenomena, the child psyche projects its thoughts towards the goal which it longs to reach. These thoughts, too, are apprehended as fixed points by the abstract conceptions of human understanding and are then concretely interpreted. The aim to be great, to be strong, to be a man, to be "above" is symbolized in the person of the father, the mother, the teacher, the coachman, the locomotive engineer, etc., and the conduct, the attitude, the imitative gestures, the play of children and their wishes, the day dreams and favorite stories, ideas about their future vocation show us that the compensatory tendency is at work and is making preparations for the future rôle. The feeling which the individual has of his own inferiority, incompetency, the realization of his smallness, of his weakness, of his uncertainty, thus becomes an appropriate working basis which, because of the intrinsically associated feelings of pleasure and pain, furnishes the inner impulse to advance towards an imaginary goal. The scheme of which the child avails himself in order to enable him to act and orient himself is one common to and in accordance with the tendency of the human understanding to reduce that which is chaotic, fluid and intangible in life to measurable entities by means of the assumption of fictions. We proceed in the same way when we divide the globe by means of meridianal and parallel lines, for thus only do we preserve fixed points which we can place in relation with each other. In all similar attempts (and the human psyche is full of them) it is the question of an introduction of an unreal and abstract scheme into actual life, and I consider the presentation of this conception as I have gathered it from the psychological observation of neuroses and psychoses and which, according to the proofs furnished by Vaihinger, manifests itself in all scientific concepts, to be the main object of this book. No matter from what angle we observe the psychic development of a normal or neurotic person he is always found ensnared in the meshes of his particular fiction; a fiction from which the neurotic is unable to find his way back to reality and in which he believes while the normal person utilizes it for the purpose of reaching a definite goal. However, that which gives such irresistible impulse to the utilization of this scheme is always the uncertainty in childhood, the great distance which separates the child from the potency of man, from the distinctions and privileges of manhood, forebodings and knowledge of which the child possesses. And in regard to this point I beg leave to supplement these statements of the learned writer, Vaihinger, namely, that the thing which impels us all and especially the neurotic and the child to abandon the direct path of induction and deduction and to use such devices as the schematic fiction originates in the feeling of uncertainty and is the craving for security, the final purpose of which is to escape from the feeling of inferiority in order to ascend to the full height of the ego-consciousness, to complete manliness, to attain the ideal of being "above." The greater the distance to this ideal, the more distinctly the guiding fiction asserts itself so that the feeling of being "under" may be just as much a determining factor as the deification of the father and mother who are the ideals of strength.

We thus see exertions put forth far beyond

those which we would expect in the most violent bodily performances which might arise from instincts, or in the strongest desire for gratification of organic longings. Goethe among others also refers to this fact that while perception is connected with the practical satisfaction of necessities, yet man carries on a life beyond this in feeling and imagination. In this thought the compulsion to the elevation of the ego-consciousness is aptly expressed, as well as in a passage occurring in one of Goethe's letters to Lavater in which he says, "This longing to elevate as high as possible the apex of the pyramid of my existence, the base of which is placed in my possession, outweighs all else and is scarcely a moment absent from thought."

It can readily be understood how such a tense psychic situation—and every artist, every genius, fights the same battle against the feeling of uncertainty; with him, however, it is the valuable cultural medium of his art—which is capable of reënforcing and bringing to light a host of traits of character which help to construct the neuroses. Thus, first of all, ambition. This is the strongest of the secondary guiding principles which strive towards the imaginary goal. And it generates a number of psychic predispositions whose purpose it is to secure to the neurotic superiority in all situations of life, but which on the other hand makes his aggressiveness, his affectivity, appear to be in a state of constant irritation. Thus the neurotic individual seems always to be proud, dogmatic, envious and miserly, seeks always to make an impression, wishes to be first, but always trembles for the result and gladly postpones decisions. Hence the hesitating, cautious behavior of neurotics, their mistrust, vacillation and doubt. As if for practice in the sense of a preliminary process he carries on these psychic preparations in small things in order to attain to fixed points and safeguarding directing principles for greater aims which hold him under their charm. This is also the meaning of Freud's displacement mechanism, i.e., the patient is impelled by his craving for security to collect proof experimentally, in *corpore vili,* which justifies and will continue to justify his entire psychic attitude. As a rule the result is always the thought, "I must be cautious, if I wish to attain my goal." And not infrequently the patient commits audaciously reckless acts in order to assure himself through an emphasis of the lesson of his recklessness the attainment of his main point, namely, the masculine ideal. Often hallucinations and dreams assume with neurotics and psychotics the function of these warning voices and depict how it has already been once before, how it has been with others, or how the thing might turn out, in order to hold the patient to the guiding principle in which he finds security.

At other times the strongly emphasized traits of eagerness for strife, obstinacy and activity, which are to "elevate" the apex of the pyramid as far as possible are strongly accentuated by pedantry which strives to keep them from changing their direction. That the eagerness for knowledge, as a mighty promoter towards attaining the high goal, is greatly overstrained, is not astonishing. With equal distinctness impatience, fear of being too late, fear of attaining nothing, manifest themselves as a particularly strong impulse to neglect no means, to do rather too much than not enough towards the attainment of the goal. These traits always lie within the field of the developed neurosis, where the feeling of "craving for security" obtrudes itself more and drives to the dangerous expedients by means of which the feeling of inferiority is rendered more profound, and the patient acts as if he were restrained, cut off from success and without hope, or he plunges to a greater or less degree into passivity, displays effeminate traits, conducts himself in a masochistic or perverse manner and finally greatly reduces his sphere of activity so that it is more shaken and more strongly dominated by the symptoms of the disease. In a similar manner arises the arrangement of indo-

lence, laziness, fatigue, impotence of every sort
which furnish a pretext to escape from decisions
which could affect the pride of the neurotic, an
excuse for withdrawing from study, from a vocation, from marriage. At times this developmental phase terminates in suicide which is then
always felt as a successful revenge on fate or on
his relatives.

Consciousness of guilt also asserts itself.
Here we find one of the most difficult points in
the analysis of neuroses and psychoses. Consciousness of guilt and conscience are fictitious
guiding principles of caution, like religiosity and
subserve the craving for security.[1] Their object
is to prevent a lowering of the ego-consciousness
when the irritated aggressiveness impels immod-
erately to selfish deeds. In the consciousness of
guilt the glance is directed backwards, conscience
operates through foresight. The love of truth,
too, is sustained by the craving for security and
belongs really within the sphere of our personal
ideal, while the neurotic lie represents a feeble
attempt to preserve appearances and to effect
compensation.

All these attempts towards elevation, efforts
of the "will to power," must naturally be understood as a form of the striving towards masculin-

[1] See Fortmuller, "Psychoanalysis and Ethics," München, E.
Reinhardt, 1912.

ity and become identified with the masculine protest, because this represents a fundamental form
of the psychical impulse to become of value, in
accordance with which all experiences, perceptions and directions of will are grouped. Apperception is guided in accordance with this most
significant scheme, namely, the goal, especially in
neurotics, is the erection of the masculine protest
against an effeminate self-estimation. Thus are
guided also attention, foresight, doubt, as well as
all traits of character and other psychic and physical inclinations, but in the highest degree and
above all the evaluation of all experiences in line
with this masculine goal, so that all these phenomena contain a dynamic which is betrayed to
the experienced, and which tends from that which
is below to that which is above, from that which
is feminine to that which is masculine. The creation of all these lines of force, the fixation of this
remote goal, the emphasis and occasional protection of inferior effeminate traits for the purpose
of combating them more forcibly by the masculine protest takes place by means of the same factor which also created the organic compensation,
i.e., the tendency towards adjustment by constant attempt to supplant an injurious, inferior
performance by an increase of effort and which in
the psychic sphere finds expression in the craving
for security which takes as a guiding line (direc-

trix) the will to power, to be manly, in order to escape the feeling of uncertainty.

The greatest difficulty which stands in the way of an understanding of the neurosis arises from the striking protection afforded these inferior, effeminate traits and their acknowledgment by the patients. Here belong all the phenomena of the disease generally, but also the passive, masochistic traits, the effeminate characteristics, the passive homosexuality, impotence, suggestibility, accessibility to and inclination for hypnosis, or, finally, the apparent surrender to effeminacy and to effeminate behavior. The final object, however, always remains the same, the domination over others which is felt and appreciated as a masculine triumph. Neither are the above described compensatory features ever absent in the makeup of these patients, as they might be expected to be in individuals who assume as a ground for action a feeling of inadequacy and who then strive to secure by every possible means a substitute for their shortcomings, to supply that which they feel to be lacking in their exaggerated ego-consciousness. And also in the psychic situation the sexual element as a symbol asserts itself, inasmuch as such patients frequently form their apperceptions in accordance with a scheme in which their genital organs are regarded as if they were effeminized, restricted, castrated, and as if they were therefore constantly forced to seek a substitute. One form of this substitution they find in the depreciation and emasculation of all other persons. From this tendency to deprive others of worth originates the considerable reënforcement of certain traits of character, which set forth further inclinations and which have the quality of injuring others, as sadism, hate, contentiousness, intolerance, envy, etc. Active homosexuality, also, as well as perversions which degrade the partner, also Lustmord, arise from the neurotic tendency to depreciate, a tendency which can hardly be pictured too strongly. They all represent a rationalization of the symbolism of subjection in line with the concept which asserts the "sexual dominance of the male." In short, the neurotic may also elevate the feeling of his own worth by degrading others.

We have mentioned above the protection of the effeminate traits in the neurosis for the purpose of better carrying on the combat, for the purpose of a better surveillance over self. These accentuations along with the distinct tendency to give preference to the will to masculinity create the appearance of a rent in the psyche of the neurotic which is familiar to writers as double personality, dissociation, and which is frequently seen in the changing humors of neurotics, but also in the succession of depression and mania, of ideas of persecution and grandeur in the psychoses. I have always found as an internal connecting bond in these antithetical conditions the tendency to maximate the ego-consciousness, whereby the "inferior" situation is associated with a degradation, but is circumscribed and arranged as a ground for operation. It is then that the masculine protest asserts itself, which is often carried to the length of asserting a resemblance to God or an intimate connection with Him. For the "splitting of consciousness" the severely schematic and very abstract process of apperception is also responsible, a form of apperception which groups the internal and external experiences according to a scheme which has the form of an absolute antithesis, something like the debits and credits in book-keeping, where there are no transitions possible. This fault of the neurotic mode of thinking, which is identical with a too far-fetched abstraction, is likewise caused by his craving for security, a tendency which requires for the purpose of making decisions, for anticipations and actions, sharply defined guiding lines, idols, false deities in which the neurotic believes. In this way he becomes estranged from concrete reality. For to find one's bearings in the world of reality an elasticity of the psyche and not a rigidity is required, a utilization of abstraction, but not an adoration, an idolizing of the same as the final purpose of existence.

Accordingly we shall find in the mental life of the neurotic, just as is the case in primitive poetry, in mythology, in legends, in cosmogony, in theogony and in the beginnings of philosophy a most pronounced tendency to give a symbolic style to himself, his experiences and to persons about him. Thus naturally the phenomena which do not belong together must be sharply separated from each other by an abstracting fiction. The impulse to this expedient arises from the longing for an orientation and has its roots in the neurotic's craving for security. This impulse is often so intense that it demands the splitting of unity, of the category, of the unity of the ego into two or more of its antithetical parts.

From the above described self-estimation of the child, who is induced by inferiority of constitution and the evils arising therefrom to strive after special securities, up to the complete development of the neurotic technique of thinking and its coadjuvant lines, of the neurotic character, a host of psychic phenomena make their appearance which according to Karl Groos [2] may be regarded as a training, according to our interpreta-

2 See Karl Groos, "Die Spiele der Menschen, Die Spiele der Thiere."

tion as a preparation for the imaginary goal. They are manifested at an early age, are indicated even in early infancy and are constantly at the foundation of the influences of conscious and unconscious education. The whole development of the child shows that it proceeds in the direction of an idea, which naturally takes a primitive form and quite regularly seeks concrete embodiment in the form of a person. Under this compulsion, the psychic mechanism of which is for the most part unconscious and only partly conscious, the psyche in the process of formation comes to more distinct expression, and the mental as well as the physical life of a human being taken at any given point of its development is to be understood as the answer which that individual gives to the question of life.

This answer, in reality the manner in which life is accepted, is according to all the knowledge thereof furnished by experience, to be considered as identical with the effort to put an end to uncertainty, to the chaos which prevails in impressions and feelings, with the effort to obtain a firm hold in order to overcome the difficulties of life. Reflection, observation, thought and forethought, attention, calculation and valuation are all efforts put forth by this craving for security. And inasmuch as the realization of one's own inferiority is taken as an abstract standard for inequality among human beings, the greater, the stronger and his measure are taken for the fictitious goal so that it may be a guarantee against this uncertainty and fright. Thus it is that the soul of the child constructs a guiding line which impels towards an elevation of the ego-consciousness in order to escape from uncertainty, the influence of which is still stronger in neurotics who have felt their inferiority more keenly. Mythographers, the human race, poets, philosophers, founders of religions have taken the material from their contemporaneous periods for the transformation of the guiding lines so that immortality, virtue, piety, riches, knowledge, social consciousness of the upper classes or self-perfection were available as goals and were utilized according to the receptive peculiarities of the individual who longed for perfection. At this point the living energies of the child become transferred into the self-created sphere of his subjective world which henceforth as a guiding fiction transmutes, falsifies and changes the values of all feelings and emotions, pleasures and pains, even the struggle for self-preservation, for his benefit, in order to attain the goal; a transformation which utilizes all the experiences of the neurotic in such a way as to bring about preparations which will ensure the triumph.

These preparatory acts with their tendency to change values may be most clearly observed in

the play of nervous children, in their delibera-
tions over the choice of a future vocation and
their physical and psychical attitudes. These
phenomena will be further discussed in connection with the dominating craving for security
which controls them. Concerning the nervous
habitus it may be stated that as a rule it is noticeable at an early age, that it takes the form of a
pantomimic representation of some trait of character, either as an anxious, waiting, distrustful,
uncertain, cautious, bashful attitude or as a hostile, obstinate, self-certain, self-complacent, forward attitude. Blushing is noticeable or the
glance is peculiarly fixed, cast down or hostile.
It is easy to correlate one of these attitudes or
gestures, or a mimic trait, with the prototype. In
nervous children imitation of the male principle,
the father, is often found; the mother only becomes a model for imitation after a formal change
in the guiding principle has taken place, or when
from the beginning the moral superiority of the
mother is beyond question. Usually these phenomena are insignificant and such as are not as
a rule subjected to the observation of the physician. Crossing the legs, the arms, a peculiar
manner of gait, preference for certain foods, bor-
rowing of certain traits of character, etc., or in
the presence of more strongly emphasized obstinacy opposite forms of expression. The re-

tained bad habits of childhood, such as eneuresis, biting the nails, sucking, stuttering, winking the eyes, masturbation, etc., can always be traced to these beginnings of obstinacy. They are the expedients of the weak to diminish the pathos of the distance and thereby do away with the feeling of inferiority, and strive in the last analysis to a transformation of authority and at the same time to gain an excuse for avoiding a decision, for postponing it.

All considerable phenomena of this sort are themselves neurotic traits of character or show that they are permeated by the neurotic character and like it itself are a form of expression of the craving for security, preparatory processes and preliminary provisions of the compensatory force which is produced by the feeling of inferiority.

CHAPTER III

THE ACCENTUATED FICTION AS THE GUIDING IDEA IN THE NEUROSIS

THE most important task of thinking is to anticipate actions or events; to seize upon an objective and ways and means and to influence them as far as possible. By means of this process of forethought, our influence over space and time is assured to a certain degree. Accordingly our psyche is first of all an organ of aggression born out of the distress of the all too restricted limitation which from the first renders difficult the gratification of natural appetites. This organically determined goal of gratification of appetites will only endure so long as the suitable means are at hand for its stabilization; for rendering it secure against the strongest attacks. Toward the end of the nursing period, when the child acquires ability to carry out independent, purposeful actions which are not merely directed toward the gratification of appetite, when he takes his place in the family and begins to adapt himself to his environment, he already possesses abilities, psychic gestures and preparations. Besides this

his conduct has acquired a certain uniformity and is seen to be on the road toward acquiring his place in the world. Such a uniformity of conduct can only be comprehended by the assumption that the child has discovered some specific fixed point outside of his own personality towards which he strives with his developmental energies. The child must, therefore, have constructed for himself a guiding principle, a guiding model, obviously in the hope of thus orienting himself in the best possible manner in his environment and of obtaining gratification of his necessities of avoiding pain and of obtaining pleasure.[1] From this guiding ideal arises the very beginning of the child's craving for tenderness, that quality which (Paulsen) originally determines the tractability of the child. Soon there become associated with this first quality, efforts to gain the praise, help and love of the parents, stirrings of independence, of obstinacy and of opposition. The child has found a meaning in life towards which he strives and whose still indistinct outlines he is forming, and starting from which he derives that quality of prevision which is calculated to direct and give worth to his actions and impulses. It is the child's helplessness, clumsiness and uncertainty which necessitates the establishment of the tentative tests of possibility, the acquisition of

[1] Adler, "Trotz und Gehorsamkeit."

experience, the creation of memories for the purpose of constructing a bridge leading to that future where there are to-be found greatness, power and satisfaction of all sorts.   The construction of this bridge is the most important work the child is called upon to perform because without it he would find himself in the midst of the inpouring impressions without order, without counsel, without guide.   It is scarcely possible to define the limits of this first stadium, of this awakening subjective world, to describe it in words.   But it may, however, be said that the guiding model of the child must be so constructed as if it were able to bring to the child greater certainty and orientation by influencing the direction of his will.

But he can only obtain security by striving towards a fixed point where he sees himself greater and stronger, where he finds himself rid of the helplessness of infancy.   The symbolic and logical nature of our process of thinking permits the construction of this future changed personality in the image of the father, the mother, of an elder brother or sister, or teacher or some professional man, or hero, or animal, or God.   The qualities of greatness, power, knowledge and ability are features common to all these guiding images and thus they are one and all symbols for imaginative abstractions.   And thus like idols made of clay they receive from the imagination of man, force and life and react upon the psyche which has created them.

This artifice of thinking would have the stamp of paranoia and of dementia precox conditions, which create for themselves hostile forces for the purpose of securing ego-consciousness, were not the child able at all times to free himself from the bonds of his fiction, to eliminate his projections (Kant) from his calculations, and to make use only of the impetus which is given him by this guiding line. His uncertainty is sufficient to make him set up a fantastic goal for the purpose of orientation in the world, but it is not so great as to make him deprive reality of its value and to assert dogmatically the reality of this guiding model, as is the case in the psychoses. One must, however, call attention to the similarity, the significance of this uncertainty and the device of a fiction in normal persons, neurotics and the insane.

The part of this process which is common to all humanity, normal and abnormal, is that the apperceiving memory is under the sway of the guiding fiction. It is because of this that there exists within certain limits in all mankind a uniformity concerning a cosmic conception. The child in its insignificance and helplessness will constantly strive to enlarge his field of power and will mark this field off after the pattern of that which seems to possess the greatest strength. And now it becomes evident in the course of psychic development that that which was at first only an imaginary expedient, important only in its relations, only a means for gaining ground to stand upon, for finding one's bearings, for gaining a foothold, has become a goal in itself, obviously because the child can only in this way obtain self-assurance in acting and not directly through the gratification of desires.[2]

Thus the effective point is found outside the corporeal sphere according to which the psyche adjusts itself, a point which forms the center of gravity of human thought, feeling and volition. And the mechanism of apperceiving memory with its host of experiences, transforms itself from an objectively operating system into a subjectively active, fictitiously modified scheme of an imagined future personality. It becomes the task of this scheme to bring about such connections with the outside world as will serve to maximate his feeling of ego-consciousness, such associations as will hint at the preparing activities and thought indicators and bring these in contact with the already existing state of preparedness. One is here reminded of the apt expression of

[2] As may be seen from Karl Groos' "Play of Animals" the understanding of the animal psyche is likewise based upon the fact that we see it act as though it were following the direction of a fictitious guiding line.

Charcot who has emphasized for science that "one only discovers that which one knows," an observation which when directed to practical experience tends to show that our whole sphere of perception is limited by a number of predetermined psychical mechanisms and predispositions as Kant's theory [3] of "a priori" forms of perception teaches us. In a similar manner our actions are determined by the content of experiences, which are given birth to and are determined by the guiding fiction. Even our judgments concerning the value of things are determined according to the standard of the imaginary goal, not according to "real" feelings or pleasurable sensations.

And conduct follows as James expresses it in consequence of a sort of approbation—depends as it were on a fiat, command or acquiescence. The guiding fiction is therefore first of all the expedient, the device by means of which the child seeks to free himself from his feeling of inferiority. It initiates compensation and stands at the service of the craving for security. The greater the feeling of inferiority, the more imperative and stronger will be the necessity for a steadying, guiding principle and indeed the more distinctly it manifests itself, and like compensa-

[3] I have to call attention here to Bergson's fundamental teachings, without being able to give room here for his important viewpoints.

tion in the organic sphere, the effectiveness of psychic compensation is linked with a functional increase and brings about novel and many-sided manifestations in the mental life. One of the forms of expression of this compensatory mechanism, intended to assure the sense of ego-consciousness is exemplified by the neurosis and psychosis.

The constitutionally inferior child with his host of disadvantages and uncertainties will construct his goal in a more definite and clearer manner, will outline more distinctly the guiding principle and will adhere to it more anxiously or dogmatically. In fact the principal impression which one gains from the observation of a neurotically disposed child is usually that the child is guided in the choice of a weapon by his somatic inferiority which he utilizes in his dealings with his relatives or which he emphasizes in his obstinacy.

Often his illness is borrowed from his environment either by simulation or exaggeration of actual ailments, all this in order to strengthen his position. Should such means not have the desired effect upon his environment, the child endeavors to rid himself of his complaints through the exercise of superior efforts, as result of which there develop not infrequently qualified and artistic performances in the event of the experiencing of an over-compensation on the part of the functional anomalies of the eye, ear, speech or musculature.   Associated with this are also stirrings of independence.   Or the remedy is sought, on the other hand, in a greater dependence, for the attainment of which, anxiety, a feeling of insignificance, weakness, awkwardness, incapacity, sense of guilt and remorse serve as strongholds. The same tendency may be seen in the adherence to the bad habits of childhood, in the retention of a psychic infantilism in so far as this is not exclusively or partially the result of obstinacy, of the infantile negativism.

A number of the complaints of psychopathic children are of a subjective nature, and correspond to a complete or partial error of judgment as it takes place in the effort of children to find a reason for their feeling of inferiority and to comprehend it.   Frequently these logical interpretations are already intermixed with the compensating ambition or with the child's aggressiveness towards its parents.   "The fault lies with my parents, with my lot, because I'm the youngest, because I was born too late, because I am a Cinderella, because I'm perhaps not the child of these parents, of this father, of this mother, because I am too small, too weak, have too small a head, am too homely, because I have an impediment of speech, a defect of hearing, am cross-eyed, nearsighted, because I have imperfect genitals, because I'm not manly, because I am a girl, because I'm bad by nature, dull and awkward, because I have masturbated, because I'm too sensuous, too covetous and naturally perverted, because I submit easily, am too dependent and obey, because I cry easily, am easily affected, because I am a criminal, a thief, an incendiary, and could murder some one. My ancestry, my education, circumcision are to blame, because I have too long a nose, too much hair, too little hair, because I am a cripple." Thus and similarly sound the child's attempts to unburden himself by blaming fate just as in the Greek fate tragedies, these are attempts to preserve the ego-consciousness and hold others responsible for his inferiority. These attempts are regularly met with in the psychic treatment of the neuroses and they can always be referred back to the relationship between an existing feeling of inferiority and an assumed ideal. The significance and value of these thought processes which are as a thorn in the side of the neurotic are noted also in the uses to which they are put by himself, first for the stimulation of his efforts in the direction of his ideal (grandiose ideas) and second, the utilization of them as a refuge and excuse when forced to a decision which threatens a lowering of the ego-consciousness (depreciatory ideas). The second applicability and application naturally occupies the foreground in the neuroses because the goal toward which the neurotic strives is set too high to be reached in a direct line. The utilization of this ideal is only rendered possible by an admixture of aggression or in blaming fate as well as heredity. By means of this the neurotic gains a permanent base of operation on the strength of which he unfolds, thrusts forward and stabilizes certain traits of character which serve the same hostile purpose, such as obstinacy, a dominating, grumbling nature, pedantry, because thereby he always succeeds in gaining mastery over his environment principally by calling attention to his terrible suffering. All of these traits and predispositions associated with bad habits retained from childhood which have become markedly exaggerated, as well as with disease symptoms of a self-created and self-modeled nature stand in the closest interrelation, are inseparable one from another and show their dependence on a factor outside their own sphere, i. e., they depend upon the guiding fiction which has evolved from the craving for security or from the longing for the maximation of the ego-consciousness. In the imaginary basis of this feeling of inferiority which because of the craving for security is always thought of in an exaggerated manner and felt too keenly, I see the chief therapeutic hope. The question whether the feeling of uncertainty is

conscious or unconscious is of secondary importance. At times pride carries things so far that
"memory gives way" (Nietzsche). Naturally
the above described connection is not realized by
the patient. It is for this reason that he remains
the plaything of his emotions and affects until
such time as the mechanism becomes revealed to
him and set to rights, until such time as the predispositions and neurotic plan of life are shat-
tered; a plaything of emotions and affects the interaction of which becomes further complicated
because of a constant admixture of traits of character intended to negate his sense of inferiority,
such as pride, envy, greed, cruelty, courage, revengefulness, irritability, etc., traits of character
which are constantly being excited through his
craving for security.

The tendency to exaggerate and emphasize
existing defects plays an important rôle in the
psychology of the neuroses. An appearance of
weakness, suffering, incapacity and uselessness
results from this manner of presenting actual defects because the neurotic is compelled by the
mechanism which controls him to conduct himself
unwaveringly in such a manner as to feel as
though he were sick, as though he were effeminate,
inferior, neglected, injured, sexually over-excited, impotent or perverted. The cautious approach to problems of life which constantly ac-

companies these impulses, the exaggerated striving upwards, the desire to play the rôle of man in some way or other, to be superior to everybody else, the neurotic's stronghold with its prime object of avoiding decisions and setbacks and thus to escape a lowering of his ego-consciousness, all of this reveals to us the true state of affairs, namely, that the low self-estimation of the neurotic is in itself an expedient by means of which he strives the more powerfully to attain that guiding goal which will bring about a maximation of his ego-consciousness. He may conduct himself according to the motto "half and half," he may cede certain strongholds in the contest but he does so solely in order to fortify himself against an ultimate feeling of inferiority and in order to be the better able to utilize others in his service.

The sexual feature of the psychology of the neuroses which Freud looks upon as a cardinal point is in this wise explained as the effect of a fiction. There is no objective standard of the "libido." The exaltation and diminution of the same is always in accord with the imaginary goal. It is easy for the neurotic to convince himself that he is the subject of a high sexual tension by means of a more or less purposeful arrangement, and especially by means of a concentration of the attention in this direction the moment he begins to seek proof of how much injury sexuality works to his feeling of security and how much his ego-consciousness is threatened from this source. The weakening of libidinous impulses even to the point of psychic impotence is to be regarded as purposeful checks on aggression, as disorders of natural predispositions, as a construction of an "as if" for the purpose of assuring himself against marriage, against a swerving from the goal, against a degradation at the hands of the sexual partner, against poverty or culpability. Repressed or conscious perverse tendencies, as well as the compulsion to masturbation are always looked upon as detours, as symbols of an imaginary plan of life whose purpose is self-assurance. They are called into being by the guiding fiction as soon as the feeling of inferiority finds expression in the fear of the sexual partner as happens regularly where there exist sexual anomalies. The fiction may then also repress the incentive to perversion into the subconscious or make the fear of the partner unrecognizable to consciousness so that it only becomes apparent from a survey of the whole situation. It resorts to the first alternative when it depends on pride for the fulfillment of its purpose, to the latter when it makes a virtue of the defect and seeks the degradation of the partner. Incestuous tendencies too, to which Freud ascribes such an important rôle in the pro-

duction of neuroses and psychoses reveal themselves in the psychology of the neuroses as purposeful edifices and symbols, which derive their
usually harmless material out of childhood life
with its preparatory processes. A proper insight
for instance into the "Œdipus complex" shows
us that it is nothing more nor less than a figurative, sexually clothed conception of what constitutes masculine self-consciousness, superiority
over woman, but at the same time betrays the
cause which leads to this phenomenon, namely as
if the mother were the only one that one could subjugate, on whom one could depend or as though
sexual desire (already in childhood) were to be
carried through in spite of everything and always
by a struggle with stronger forces (the father,
dragons, danger of death). As may be inferred
from this interpretation, close inquiry into the
sexual neuroses always leads to the discovery of a
guiding fiction which reveals itself in a sexual
form or can be revealed by therapeutists, as well
as to the laying bare of a mode of apperception
evolved according to a sexual scheme in consequence of which the neurotic and often also the
normal person attempt to apprehend and understand the world and all its phenomena in sexual
terms, in a sexual picture as it were. Our further
investigations reveal that this sexual scheme
which is often carried out in speech, in custom,

and manners, is only a variation of that all-embracing scheme of more fundamental origin, i.e., the antithetical mode of apperception as "male-female" "up-down." [4] The later psychic perverse tendencies derive their material and impulse from the harmless bodily sensations and misjudgments of childhood which when occasion arises are given an extraordinarily high value or some chance pleasurable sensations are perceived as analogues of sexual sensations. The psychologist must not assume the same point of view, must not maintain such a mode of apperception as valid, not substitute real sexual components for a fiction as the patient does. His task on the contrary consists in revealing to the patient the superficiality of his attempts at orientation, to tear it apart as mere product of the imagination, and to weaken the feeling of inferiority which drives the patient in a convulsive manner towards these guiding principles which would necessitate the carrying out of the "masculine protest" in a circuitous manner.

Apperceiving memory which influences our

[4] See the dream of Hippias, Herodotus VI, 107; "he dreamt that he was sleeping with his mother." This he dreamed as he was about to conquer his maternal city, as he had already done once before as the companion of his father. Thus the Œdipus complex as the symbol of the desire to dominate. With the Romans too Beischlaf (sexual congress) symbolized conquest, victory. Compare the double meaning of the word "subigere."

cosmic picture to such a great extent works also with a fiction as it were, with a schematic fiction, in accordance with which we choose and model our perceptions, our experiences, as well as the training of all our connate tendencies and capacities until they are changed into the appropriate psychical and technical skillfulness and preparedness. The modus operandi of our conscious and unconscious memory and its individualization obey the personal ideal and its standards. From this we are able to deduce that as a guiding fiction its purpose is to confront the problems of life so soon as the feeling of inferiority and uncertainty impels toward compensation. This fixed guiding point of our efforts, which in no sense possesses reality, is absolutely decisive for the psychic development, for it enables us to make steps in the chaos of the world, as does the child when learning to walk and keeping in his eye a goal which he strives to reach. Far more unwaveringly, the neurotic keeps before his eye his God, his idol, his ideal of personality and clings to his guiding principle, losing sight in the meanwhile of reality, whereas the normal person is always ready to dispense with this crutch, this aid, and reckon unhampered with reality. In this instance, the neurotic resembles a person who looks up to God, commends himself to the Lord and then and there awaits credulously for his guidance; he is nailed to the cross of his fiction. The normal individual too may and does create his deity, feels drawn upward but never loses sight of reality, and always takes it into account as soon as he is called upon to act. Accordingly the neurotic lives under the hypnotic influence of an imaginary plan of life.

That this imaginary mark of the personal ideal situated as it is beyond space and time is never without effect, may be seen from the trends of the attention; interests and tendencies of these individuals, which always lead to points of view of an a priori nature. The exquisite purposefulness of our psychic processes and the predisposition determined thereby is responsible for the fact that our actions have definite beginnings and terminations, that, as Ziehen emphasizes, voluntary and involuntary actions are constantly aimed at attaining a definite result, that we must assume with Pawlow a decided intelligence in the functioning of the organs. All these phenomena are so convincing that philosophers and psychologists have from the earliest times taken as a teleologic dogma everything which premeditatively attempted an orientation according to an assumed fixed point as the goal.

The concept of natural selection is entirely too inadequate to explain results which are able to take on new and changing forms as occasion demands. Experience compels us to consider all these phenomena as dependent upon an unconsciously active fiction, the faint conscious irradiations of which furnish us goals, according to which in the last analysis our apperception of all our experiences and activities is shaped. It is less difficult to prove the details of this guiding fiction, than the fiction itself, than the fictitious goal itself. Psychological research has called attention to various such goals. For our purpose it will suffice to consider critically just two of these. Most authorities content themselves with the view that all human activity, all volition is dominated by feelings of pleasure and pain. Upon superficial consideration these authors seem to be correct in their assumptions, because as a matter of fact the human psyche does tend to seek pleasure and avoid pain. But the foundation of this theory is unstable. There is no standard for feelings of pleasure, indeed no standard for feeling at all. There exists furthermore no perception, no action, the effect of which may not vary in accordance with place and time, under some circumstances causing pleasure; under others pain. And even the primitive sensations resulting from satisfaction of organic desires have their gradations and vary with the degree of satiability and in accordance with cultural guiding principles, so that for satisfaction in itself to serve as the goal, it requires extreme denial, and abstinence. Now granting that satisfaction has actually been attained, does the psyche really lose its directing principle? The psyche's iron necessity for orientation and security requires for their establishment and their functions a more stable standpoint than the vacillating and uncertain principle of gratification of desire, and a more stable point of view than the object of attaining gratification. The impossibility of orienting one's self and one's actions according to such a goal forces even the child to abandon efforts in this direction. Finally it is a misuse of an abstraction to single out and emphasize by means of a petitio principii, out of the various complex psychic activities, the quest of pleasure, as the motive force, after every isolated impulse has already been explained—as pleasure seeking, as libidinous. Shiller with a keenness of vision trained in the school of Kant saw much further when he made a place in the coming "philosophy" for the directing influence of earthly events, and even went so far as to consider it (philosophy) dependent on "hunger and love."

To ascribe, however, the whole directing force to sexuality as Freud does, or what is for him the same thing, to the libido, to ascribe this whole influence to nothing but love is a violation of logical thinking itself, a fiction of a bad sort, which when accepted as a dogma must lead to great contradictions and confusion of concepts because it contrasts altogether too much with reality.

The disapproval of the principle of "self-preservation" is more difficult, especially as that principle is supported on the one hand by arguments of a teleological significance, on the other hand by the import of Darwin's theory of natural selection. But we see constantly that we undertake courses of action contrary to the principles of self-preservation or to the preservation of the species, yes, that a certain arbitrariness (Fres-Meyerhof) permits us, in regard to self-preservation as well as in regard to pleasure, to raise or lower our valuations, that we often wholly lose sight of self-preservation when pleasure or pain enter into the question, and that on the other hand we often sacrifice pleasure when an injury is threatened to the ego. In what manner do these two incentives which are certainly not without influence, range themselves under the main guiding principle which impels to the elevation of the ego-consciousness? The two points of view correspond to two types of individuals (to which it is possible to add still others) one of which is least able to dispense with pleasure in his ego-consciousness, while the other places first importance on the feeling of life, on the feeling of immortality. Therefore, there arise modified modes of perception which produce antitheses in thought in the sense of "pleasure—pain" or "life—death." The former are unable to deprive pleasure of value, the latter life. In the sense of procreation which is again thought of in the manner of the antithetical scheme "male-female," these two types approach each other and seek expression in the direction of the masculine protest. As far as neurotics are concerned the one type has always sought to compensate the painful feeling of his somatic inferiority, the other type has grown up in the fear of death, of dying early. Their view of the world furnishes them only fragments, their soul is partially color-blind, but notwithstanding this often more keen-sighted than the Daltonists in their understanding of color.

We close this critical observation with a reference to the absolute principle of the "will to power" a guiding fiction which sets in more forcibly and earlier, and is precipitated and matured, in proportion to the prominence assumed by the consciousness of inferiority in the physically inferior child. The ideal of personal importance as a point toward which all efforts are directed is created by the craving for security and contains as imaginary qualities all the powers and natural gifts of which the child believes himself deprived. This fiction, more exaggerated than under normal conditions, molds the mentality, the traits of character and predispositions in its own image.

The neurotic apperception proceeds according to a figurative scheme containing sharply opposed antitheses, and the grouping of the impressions and emotions takes place according to correspondingly false and imaginary values.

It lies in the nature of the neurotic fiction, of the exaggerated idea of personal worth, to reveal itself under two forms, sometimes as an "abstract mechanism" sometimes as a concrete picture, or as a phantasy, as an idea. In the first case the connection of what is symbolic in the representation with the compensated feeling of inferiority should not be lost sight of, and in the second case one must above all take into consideration the decisive share in the process taken by the psychic dynamic which impels "upwards." [5] In the analysis of a psychogenic disease so long as the guiding tendency "upwards" does not reveal itself, the nature of the disease remains hidden to us, for no matter how valuable the insights of the psycho-therapeutists have been, so long as the secondary guiding principle of attaining pleasure, of affectivity (Bleuler) and those which originate as result of physical inferiority (Adler) are not referred back to the ideal of personality—our understanding remains imperfect, "there is still unfortunately lacking the psychic bond." It is also

[5] Of the later authors who have especially emphasized this point of view, I must especially mention H. Silberer.

not astonishing that in different cases different characteristics are given to this ideal of personality and usually various characteristics at one and the same time as these are derived from various sorts of organ defects, usually from several at the same time. A preliminary, decidedly incomplete diagram which would correspond more to the "abstract psyche" of the neurotic than to that of the normal individual would be the following:

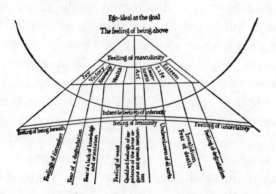

In this outline the most varied combinations must be imagined, if it is to serve its purpose as a model for the purpose of superficial orientation. Instead of discussing these combinations and the multitudinous components we will discuss some distinguishing phenomena which seem important for the understanding of the neuroses and the neurotic character.

Each of the abstract guiding lines of the neurosis and of its underlying psychic mechanism may become accessible to consciousness by means of a memory-picture or may be rendered accessible to it. This picture may originate from the remnants of a childhood experience, or it is a product of phantasy, a species of the craving for security. It may represent a symbol, a trade-mark as it were, for a certain mode of reaction, now and then reaching development or being reformed only at a later period often when the neurosis is already fully developed. Being obviously the effect of a sort of economy of thought, which is furnished by the principle of least resistance (Avenarius), it is never of consequence as far as its content is concerned, but only as an abstract scheme or as the remnant of a psychic experience in which the will to power once filled its destiny. This schematic fiction, no matter how concretely it may manifest itself, is never to be understood otherwise than in an allegorical sense. In it is reflected an actual constituent part of experience together with a "moral" both of which are retained by memory in the interest of the self-assurance that is aimed at, either as a memento, to adhere more tenaciously to the guiding principle or as a fore-judgment not to abandon it. None of these memory pictures has ever had pathogenic significance, like a psychic trauma for in-

stance, and it is only when the neurosis super-
venes, when the feeling of degradation of the ego-
consciousness leads to the masculine protest and
because of this to a closer attachment to the already long established compensatory guiding
principles are these memory pictures hunted out
from material belonging to a remote past and
come to light because of their usefulness, partly
in order to make possible the neurotic's conduct
and partly to give it meaning. Here belong
above all pain, anxiety and affect predispositions
which are based upon such reminiscences which
may become actualized in an hallucinatory manner, and which may be likened to visual and auditory hallucinations. Naturally those reminiscences will be typical which stand in the closest
possible relation to the guiding principle because
they represent or simulate for the neurotic, clinging as he does to the guiding principle, both the
greater and smaller detours of which he has
to avail himself in order to elevate his ego-consciousness. The characteristic of the neurotic
psyche is only its tenacious adherence to the guiding principle.   It is the contradictions with reality, the conflicts which arise from them and the
urgency to acquire social importance and power,
which bring forth the symptoms. This is even
more obvious in such psychoses where the guiding
principle appears most subtly. Misinterpreta-

tions of reality are undertaken, and demonstrations result, merely, so to speak, for the sake of proof. In both instances, the patient behaves as though he had the goal constantly before his eyes. In the case of the neurosis he exaggerates and combats the real obstacles to the maximation of his ego-consciousness or seeks to avoid them by the construction of excuses. The psychotic individual clinging as he does to his idea (fixe idée) seeks to ignore reality or to transform it in such a way as to make it correspond with his unreal standpoint. Freud, who has done so much toward the discovery of symbolism in the neurosis and psychosis, has called attention to the galaxy of symbols. Unfortunately he has carried his investigations only to the point of discovering the actual or possible sexual formulæ in these symbols, and has not pursued their further elucidation into the dynamic eventuality of the masculine protest, of striving "upward." Thus it happened that for him the meaning of the neurosis became exhausted in the conversion of libidinous stimuli whereas, in reality that which lies behind the symbolism is the appearance of or the actual impulsion toward a maximation of the masculine ego-consciousness.

We have described the guiding ideal of the ego as a fiction, thus denying its reality, but we must nevertheless assert that although unreal it is of the greatest importance for the process of life, and for the psychic development. Vaihinger in his "Philosophy of As If" has given a brilliant elucidation of this apparent contradiction, and recognized the fiction as an opposition to reality but as indispensable for the development of science. Reference to this singular relationship in the psychology of the neuroses was first made by me and I was considerably assisted and confirmed in my view by Vaihinger's work. I am thus in a position to say something concerning the fiction of ego-consciousness, and to throw some light on its significance as well as on its mode of appearance in the psyche. It is first of all an abstraction and must in itself be regarded as the indication of an anticipation. It is, so to speak, the marshall's staff [6] in the wallet of the insignificant soldier, and may be looked upon as "payment on account" demanded by the primitive feeling of uncertainty. The construction of the fiction takes place by setting aside disquieting inferiorities and burdensome realities in the idea, as always happens when the psyche seeks

[6] For the benefit of psychologists of a keener insight, I note here that the prevalence of examples which have been taken from military life have been chosen by me with an especial object in view. In military training the starting point and fictive purpose are brought into closer relation, can be more readily noted, and every movement of the training soldier becomes a dexterity which has for its purpose the transformation of a primary feeling of weakness into a feeling of superiority.

certainty and escape from its restraint. The painful uncertainty is reduced to its lowest possible, albeit apparently causal amount, and this is transformed into its very antithesis which is in turn made into the fictive goal of every wish-phantasy and desire. It is then that this goal may be made concrete for the sake of becoming self-evident. For instance, the restriction of food in childhood is felt as an abstract "nothing," as want, in contrast to this feeling the child comes to long for "all," for superfluity until it brings this goal much nearer to the understanding in the person of the father, in the form of a traditionally rich person, of a mighty Kaiser. The more intensely the deprivation was felt the more forcible is this imaginary abstract ideal constructed and starting therefrom begins the formation and classification of the given psychical forces to preparatory attitudes, facilities and traits of character. The individual then carries these traits of character demanded by the fictive goal just as the mask of the ancient actor—persona—was required to fit to the dénouement of the tragedy. Should there stir in a boy doubt concerning his manliness, as happens in constitutionally inferior children, feeling as they do to be kindred to girls, he chooses a goal of such a nature as will give him mastery over women (usually also over all men). Through this his attitude toward women is determined at an early age. He will constantly show a tendency to bring about his superiority over women, will undervalue and degrade the feminine sex, will, figuratively speaking—raise the hand against his mother, which in neurotically disposed children often finds expression in a gesture or in their psychic attitude, and will in a playful manner take his model from the mother in order to test himself in the manly rôle before it. The development of this sort of infantile attitude of readiness where a rigid pedantic behavior becomes manifest, where the child's excited desire for mastery seeks a confirmation, and an assurance of his ego-consciousness, similar to the one he has experienced from his mother, that is, conditions in which he is able in the same manner to satisfy his craving for security is already to be looked upon as a neurotic trait. It is only to this neurotic fixity of the uncertainty that Nietzsche's assertion is applicable, namely that "every one carries within him a portrait of womankind which he has derived from his mother, and which makes him honor woman or despise her or entertain a total indifference toward her." Yet we must concede that these individuals are in the majority. Among them are many who were disdained by their mother, since which time they fear a like setback from every woman, or demand from her an extraordinary measure of surrender.

In the life and development of man there is nothing that sets to work with greater secrecy than the construction of the ideal of personality. If we inquire into the cause of this secrecy, it seems that the most important basis lies in the combative, not to say hostile character of this fiction. It has originated through a constant measuring and weighing of the advantages of others and must therefore bring about according to the principle of antithesis which lies at the root of this process, the injury to others. The psychological analysis of the neurotic shows always the presence of the tendency to depreciation, which is summarily directed toward every one. The combative tendencies [7] become regularly manifest in greed, in envy, in longing for superiority. But the fiction of gaining the mastery over others can only be used, be taken into account if it does not disturb the combination of relations from the beginning. And therefore, this fiction must early become unrecognizable, must assume a disguise, or it destroys itself. This disguise takes place by the positing of an anti-fiction, which first of all directs visible conduct, and under the stress of which reality is ap-

[7] S. "Der Aggressionstrieb im Leben und in der Neurose."

proached, and the recognition of its effective forces is accomplished. This contrary fiction, always of the nature of current, corrective instances, brings about the formal change of the guiding fiction by pressing its own claim to consideration, by presenting for recognition social and ethical demands at their true value and thus assuring the reasonableness of thinking and acting. It is the security coefficient of the guiding line to power and the harmony of the two fictions, their mutual compatibility which is the sign of mental health. In the contrary fiction are active experience and education, social and cultural formulas, and the traditions of society. In times of good humor, of security, of normal conditions, of peace, this is the prevailing form, which causes a restraint of the combative predispositions and effects an adaptation of the traits of character to the environment. Should the insecurity increase and the consciousness of inferiority emerge, then the contrary-fiction is deprived of value because of an increasing abstraction from reality, the dexterities become mobilized, the nervous dogmatic character asserts itself and with it the exaggerated sense of ego-ideal. It is one of the triumphs of human wit to put through the guiding fiction by adapting it to the antifiction, to shine through modesty, to conquer by humility and submissiveness, to humiliate

performances of the neurotic psyche. The over-tense personal ideal, however, which acquires absolute rigidity, which assumes nearly an identity with God, often lends to the nature and behavior of the neurotic and psychotic a pronounced hypomanic character, if the preparations therefore, the feeling of insignificance, the ideas of persecution did not counteract this character by causing a sort of inner certainty without which the positing of the goal would be impossible, by causing a feeling of predestination. In the phases of greater insecurity this characteristic is considerably stronger and its significance as anticipation of the guiding fiction, as payment on account becomes distinctly obvious.

Gustav Freytag in his "Reminiscences of my Life" describes the usefulness of the compensatory performance in the following manner:

"But too the bull's-eye-shot on the target is difficult to me. For at Oels I had noticed during the instruction that I was very near sighted. When I complained of this during the vacation to my father, he advised me to make my way through the world without glasses and told me a story illustrating the helplessness of a theologist who had made him get up out of bed one morning to hunt his spectacles so that he could find his trousers. I followed this advice and have accustomed myself to the use of spectacles only at the

theater and in looking at pictures. I sought to
overcome the disadvantages under which I la-
bored in society from this defect and overlooked
much unsuspectedly which would have disgusted
a sharper observer. I was often obliged to
forego the enjoyment of flowers, beauty in dress,
of remarkable countenances and beauty in women
from which others derived pleasure. But as the
same adjusted itself adroitly to this defect of
sense, there was soon developed in me a good understanding of those expressions of life which
came within my range of vision and a quick divi-
nation of much which was not clear to me; the
smaller number of the perceptions permitted me
to elaborate those which were perceived with
greater ease and perhaps more profoundly. At
any rate the loss was greater than the gain. But
my father was thus far right, my eyes preserved
unchanged throughout my entire life their keenness of vision at close distances."

If one imagines the development of a visual
phantasy of this sort which constantly draws
away from reality goaded by the pressure of the
craving for security, there results for the same
purpose of obtaining security as in the above
cited example, an ability to produce visual hallucinations which can manifest itself even outside
of dream states, for the purpose of presenting
warnings to preserve personal security and en-

couraging consolations. The abstractions and also the anticipations have even gone farther and may lead to the well known remarkable pathological expressions of the "telepaths" or Cassandra natures. The disquieting consciousness of inferiority gives a terrible incentive to this reaching out beyond the limits of human possibilities here as in other instances, and this consciousness finding refuge in weakness ascribes to others a greater power of vision, as though they could see what was hidden, could read the thoughts. The child in his craving for security with his natural secrecy may early incline to just this point in order to gain security, and act under the imaginary assumption that others can "see into his heart," can divine his most hidden thoughts, an assumption which often makes its appearance as an expedient in the neurosis and psychosis and has the same value as the exaggerated feeling of guilt, perhaps, and neurotic conscientiousness, and whose purpose is to avoid a degradation of self-esteem, shame, punishment, mockery, humiliation, the feminine rôle, death.

The increased capacity of the neurotic for abstractions for anticipations is not only at the root of his hallucinatory character, of his fantasies and his dreams but also of the over-exertion of organ functioning of which he makes use in purposeful efforts as preparations for the combat.

Thus the neurotic makes for himself a place by more abstract prevision and premeditation, and constructs thereof, that neurotic foresight which is regularly present in this disease, by means of which the patient holds the possibilities of experience constantly before him arranged dogmatically and in sharply antithetical groups according to the Scheme "Triumph—Defeat." Or he places his environment under ban by heightening the sensibility of his organs (which is the first step towards hallucinations) showing hypersensibility to smells, sounds, touch, temperature, tastes and pains, and this brings his undertakings constantly into harmony with his imaginary masculine guiding principle. Foolishness and superstitious convictions of a hopeless destiny, the firm seated belief in one's own ill luck serve the same purpose of satisfying the craving for security by constructing the proof that caution is necessary. The hallucinatory awakening of anxiety works in the same direction, of which the neurotic makes extensive use.

That the traits of character as well as the emotional predispositions serve the guiding fiction, it is the purpose of this book to prove to the fullest degree. The guiding line of the neurotic leading in a directly perpendicular line upwards demands peculiar expedients and forms of life which are included under the little uniform concept of the neurotic symptoms. Now one finds safety-devices at remote places, prohibitory arrangements, protective combats, for the purpose of assuring success to the central impulse, the will to power, then again there are, and these are often difficult to understand, circuitous ways comparable to secret paths, taken so as not to lose the guiding line when the direct way to the masculine triumph is barred. Often a change of nervous phenomena is observed which resembles tentative experiments, until the more severe symptom guarantees a concordance with the guiding idea.

I believe too that I have presented in the present work these symptoms and their psychogenesis coherently and to a sufficient extent. They all rest on dexterity acquired by long practice and preparation whose hypervalency is supported through the medium of and is founded on the fitness for the combat to preserve the ideal self-esteem. The preparations themselves commence in the beginning of the neurosis, accompany the development of the idea of personal worth and are adapted to it. They are most clearly recognized in the reminiscences of childhood which have been presented in the oft returning dreams, in the mimic, the habitus, in the play of children, in their phantasies, concerning future vocations, concerning the future.

It lies in the nature of the too elevated guiding

idea that it should estrange the person who entertains it, that is the neurotic, from reality.
Not infrequently this condition manifests itself
in a "feeling of strangeness" which is again over-
estimated and used with a view to a certain effect,
i.e., to recommend a cautious retreat in an insecure situation. Apparently opposite to this
"back" an unjustified feeling of confidence in a
situation, the feeling of "deja vu" sometimes becomes manifest, often in the form of a concealed
analogy for the purpose of warning or encouraging.[8]   In neurotic students I have sometimes observed that led by the feeling of their predestination scholars have sought a hearing on subjects
with which they were wholly unfamiliar with the
result of total failure.   Such experiences may
cause the neurotic to be suspicious of his emphasized feeling of "self-confidence" which may
emerge, as though he preserved a bad after-taste.
The security through the exaggerated idea of
self-esteem and the adherence to it determines
often the feeling of or even a real condition of
estrangement from the world, which indeed is
usually exaggerated with a definite purpose.
Fear for everything now, ponderousness, awk-

[8] The feeling of strangeness and the feeling of familiarity in
the neurosis are analogous to the image of warning and exhortation
of an inner voice in the dream, the hallucination and the attitude in
the psychosis.

wardness, bashfulness, then accompany the neurotic who avoids reality and reveals his efforts to
reinterpret, reconstruct and remodel it.   This
deficiency also seeks its compensation and in less
severe cases finds it in the antifiction leading to
reality, which again in an abstract, usually urgent
form seeks to over-estimate the significance of
the reality from exaggerated fear of it in order
to raise up preparations against error and defect
at all times.   The vacillation between the ideal
and the real manifests itself in an extreme way
in the neurotic psyche, in which the passion for
doubting assumes the form of a paradigm for the
real "truth," as the final goal of power which
the neurotic is to attain.   Or the outer forms are
pedantically held to and over-estimated as is a
fetish, and as though they guaranteed security.
The following sentence from Hebel's letters [9]
seems to me to indicate this feature.

"One can never pay sufficient honor to the
outer forms which in youth are so thoughtlessly
ridiculed, for they are the only lines which assist
in making decisions in the restlessly changing
world without law or order"—   In small things
as in great this craving for security is always
manifested and humanity is always seeking it by
analogies, and by abstract dogmatic methods.

[9] R. W. Werner, from Hebel's youth, Oesterreichische Rundschau, 1911.

The frequency of sexual guiding lines in the neuroses is explained in unprejudiced analyses upon the following grounds:

1. Because they furnish a suitable form of expression for the masculine protest.

2. Because it lies within the option of the patient to feel them as real.

Therefore, the adaptation of the sexual imaginary guiding line depends also on its value in procuring security for the feeling of self-esteem, on its significance as an abstraction and quality of exciting hallucinations, and on its quality of easily receiving a concrete form and because it admits of anticipations.

According to this the hallucinatory character of the neurotic is a peculiar instance of the mechanism of security. It makes use, as does thinking and speech, of the primitive recollections reduced to the smallest dynamic measure to which he is drawn by means of the abstracting power of the craving for security. Its function and office is to calculate the way to the desired heights by use of analogy from experiences which have their place in childhood in emphasizing set-backs that have been endured or comforting memories of evils that have been overcome.

The hallucinatory power represents a completed preparation accomplished by the overstrained craving for security, and takes its material, as does also the function of thought and premeditation from the cast-iron element of the neurotically directed memory. That which is called regression in dream and in hallucinations by other writers is the every-day process of thought which gropes back to experience, and can only refer to the material of the dreams and hallucinations, but never to their dynamics.

The psychic dynamic of an hallucination consist therefore in this, that in a situation of uncertainty, a guiding line is sought with might and is hypostasized by means of an abstraction, per analogium with the evaluation of experience, by means of anticipation and by means of a fictitious rendition of something closely related to a sensory perception. This latter ability as the most effective means of expression may, by reason of the anti-fiction which inclines to reality, be felt as in conscious opposition to reality as in dreams, or in the craving for security dissolves the anti-fiction and permits the hallucination to be felt as real.

Jodl defined civilization as "the increased effort of man under certain circumstances and with special intensity to secure his person and life against hostile powers of nature as well as from the antagonism of his fellow men, to satisfy his needs both real and ideal in a greater measure and to bring his nature without obstacle to development."

The neurotic individual holds the guiding line much more constantly in view, but may accordingly need to bring to expression schematically and dogmatically the guiding line which leads to the transcendental or the anti-fiction which tends to culture, the latter in the sense of a neurotic circuitous way, in which, for example, he seems to submit to an extreme degree to the "antagonism of his fellow men" for the purpose of triumphing over them.

The evolution of the effort to bring his nature to the fullest development, to attain the pinnacle of that which the neurotic individual may call his culture leads us back again to the already mentioned preparations so important from a psychological point of view, to the tentative efforts which are supposed to be introduced by the original consciousness of inferiority.

All the imperfect organs in a state of infantile development strive with all their connate capacities and possibilities of development to form purposeful, so to speak intelligent preparatory arrangements. In the efforts of the constitutionally inferior organs with their numerous abortive performances arises, as a consequence of the greater tension in the presence of the requirements of the external world, the impression of uncertainty, the self-esteem of the child brings forward a permanent consciousness of inferiority.

Thus it happens that already in early childhood the mastery of the situation according to an example taken as a model or to dominate the situation even far beyond the power indicated in the model is taken as the guiding motive and a permanent impulse of will is founded which hands over the permanent guidance to a directing idea —"the will to power." The positing of a goal in the neurotic character is a phase of the same tendency. This goal corresponds consciously or unconsciously to the formula: "I must act in such a way that in the end I become the master of the situation." Long continuation of the child in the phase of consciousness of inferiority leads to a heightening and strengthening of the intensity of that formula, so that from the unusual intensity of all efforts, the preparatory actions and the predispositions, the traits of character of any period of development may be inferred as original consciousness of inferiority. Also in organs falling below the normal standard the tentative efforts are manifested, which produce preparations and expedients in walking, seeing, eating, hearing. Exner emphasizes that these tentative efforts are like those which precede the grasping of the sound combinations when children are learning to speak. Much more convulsive in form are the preliminary processes in the defective organ, whose preparations and methods of functioning in favorable examples of over-compensation, are in height, light artistic performances and perfection, but which often as in the neurosis because of the close guard kept and the cautiousness, rarely attain full development. The child seeks to learn his faults in the way offered him by the craving for security, and seeks to remedy them or to gain advantage from them in using them as an expedient. As he does not know the real reason for his inferiority, often from pride does not wish to know them, he is easily misled to ascribe them to external reasons, to blame the "spits of objects" or usually, his relatives, and assumes then an aggressive, hostile attitude to the real objective world. Usually he retains a foreboding, a presentiment of ill-luck as an abstract reminder of his feelings of inferiority, which he is likely to exaggerate, often develops to a feeling of guilt, if circumstances admit of this, in order to unfold his pre-vision, his foresight with good reason. The neurotic endeavors are above all directed towards enlarging and securing the boundaries of self-esteem by constantly estimating and testing the powers in the difficulties of the objective world.

To over-exertion in this effort may be traced many of the traits of the neurotic—his inclination to play with fire, to make dangerous situations and hunt for them, his pleasure in the gruesome and the diabolical (Michel). The inclination to crime, like the sadistic inclination lies in the masculine guiding line, but is often neutralized by the contradictory idea which develops and is more often exaggerated in memory, with the purpose of warning from execution.

Nervousness, by preference, utilizes organic defectiveness, the infantile defects, the sense of ill-health in general, on the one hand for the purpose of securing the ego-consciousness against the requirements of parental authority, usually by means of a stubborn revolt on the other hand for the purpose of postponing by a sort of artificial obstruction decisions and collisions which might be dangerous to the masculine fiction, that is to say, the relinquishing of certain positions of advantage in order to retain more important ones. Indeed the neurotic individual often seeks minor defeats, even brings them about artificially, or assumes dangerous outlooks in order thereby to justify his neurotic acts and caution. In neurotically retained childhood defects a special refractoriness and strong aggression against the father and mother may be expected.

Thus a compulsory striving toward the understanding of objective difficulties, efforts to overcome them, to gain the mastery, to combat them, undervaluation and depreciation of life and its joys or flight from them characterize a phase of the neurosis. Along with this the fact very frequently comes to light that the patient is very enthusiastic for life, for work, for love and marriage, but platonically, while secretly he bars the access to them through the neurosis, in order to make sure of his domination in the more limited field of the family with the father and mother.

This outwardly directed anxious and cautious glance of the neurotic which is intended to preserve the guiding fiction is regularly accompanied by a self-observation of a higher intensity. Sometimes in a situation of psychic uncertainty the personified, deified guiding idea is met with as a second self, as an inner voice like the Dæmon of Socrates which warns, encourages, punishes, accuses. And that which the neurasthenics and hypochondriacs relate to us concerning the manner in which they inwardly rage, how keenly they examine and follow every act of their lives is true of neurotics generally. The self-observation may lead to a limitation of the field of combat, through it it utilizes expressions of fear of sickness, by means of which the neurotic individual is always in a position to beat a retreat for the sake of security. It must be thought of as effective, when the primitive expedients for gaining security, such as anxiety, shame, bashfulness, or the more complex ones, as modesty, conscientiousness, nervous attacks, accompany the presentiment of a defeat, in order not to allow the self-esteem to sink below the required level. Self-observation and self-esteem always excited and reënforced by the guiding fiction so that a base of operation is offered and the aggressions introduced produce immediately the neurotic, dogmatic traits of character, of envy, greed, tyranny, etc. The exaggerated introspection plays a constant rôle in the continuous measuring and wrestling of the neurotic individual to test his own worth against that of others, it gives hints to premeditation and phantasy and announces its presence when the patient avoids making a decision or when for the same purpose he gives himself up permanently to doubt.

That all these introspections originate from the feeling of insufficiency and are influenced by it is just as easy to understand, as that they finally reach the goal to which they in reality tend, i.e., caution. Thus introspection is at once hesitation, egotism, megalomania, doubt, self-depreciatory psychosis, and stands in connection with all other phenomena which are caused by the consciousness of inferiority. It serves especially for the reënforcement and testing of the masculine protest, of characteristics such as courage, pride, ambition, etc., as well as the purpose of increasing all those tendencies whose acme is security, such as economy, exactness, industry, cleanliness.

It influences the attention and serves also to dominate it, so that it occupies a prominent position in that mesh of traits whose object it is to gain security. The results, however, at which it arrives are purposely falsified. It would be very erroneous to regard it as libidinous or as pleasure producing. Its function is rather to group all the impressions of the objective world and to bring them under a single test, in such a way, so to speak, that the primary uncertainty of the individual shall be assured from being unmasked by a mathematical or statistical guarantee according to the standard of probability, i.e., that the individual shall escape a defeat. I first called attention to the dynamic of the neurosis in the "Neurotic Disposition" and the object of the present work is to present it in a more profound and extended form. The purposeful and profound introspection, therefore, is in line with the neurosis, even though in philosophy, psychology and in self-knowledge it has produced excellent fruit. It is the private philosophy of the neurotic which fails to hit the mark of reality, and whose mania, corrigible by analysis, has its analogy in the "know thyself" of the sublime philosophers. The largely incorrigible delirium of the psychotics brooding and phantastic introspection, which is so much easier to comprehend as a systematized illusion with the object of assuring self-esteem, teaches us to understand the delirium of the introspection of the neurotic.

The neurotic's striving for security, his very stronghold, can therefore only be understood when the original, contrary factor of his uncertainty is likewise taken into consideration. Both are the result of an antithetically grouped judgment which has come to depend on the fictitious egotistic ideal, which furnishes to this judgment biased "subjective" values. The feeling of "security" and its opposite pole of "insecurity" arranged according to the antithesis of "feeling inferiority" and "egotistic ideal" are like these latter a fictitious pair of values, a psychic formation of which Vaihinger says "that the real in them is artificially placed there, that only when taken together have they meaning and value, taken singly, however, they lead through their isolation to nonsense, contradictions and illusionary problems. In the analysis of psychoneuroses it always becomes obvious that this antithesis resolves itself in accordance with the only real "antithesis" of "man—woman," so that the feeling of inferiority, uncertainty, lowliness, effeminacy, falls on one side of the table, the antithesis of certainty, superiority, self-esteem, manliness, on the other. The dynamics of the neurosis can therefore be regarded (and is often so understood by the neurotic because of its irradiation upon his psyche) as if the patient wished to change from a woman to a man.   This effect yields in its most highly colored form the picture of that which I have called the "masculine protest."

The strength of the manly element in the idea of cultural perfection as well as more particularly in the artificial guiding lines of neurotics as we find it in the wishes and actions, thoughts and feelings of our patients, in their attitude toward the objective world, in their preparations for life, in every trait of character, in every physical and psychical gesture, which gives the impulse to the upward movement and directs the line of life upward, permits us to divine that in the beginning of psychical development a deficiency of such manly power was felt, and that the original feeling of inferiority realized by the constitutionally defective child was estimated as feminine in conformity with this antithesis.   No matter what was at the foundation of the feeling of inferiority, when the strong neurotic stronghold is introduced through the setting up of the masculine fiction, the supposed basis of the childish uncertainty and the uncertainty itself fall under the phenomena which are considered as effeminate as a consequence of the neurotic, antithetical grouping.   The feeling of insignificance, of weakness, of anxiety and helplessness, of ill health, of deficiency, of pain, etc., produces in the neurotic actions of such a nature that he seems to be compelled to set up a defense against effeminacy, that is to say, to be obliged to act in a manly and forceful manner. In the same manner this answer follows, the affect-possibilities of the masculine protest react against every degradation, against the feeling of uncertainty, of being injured, of inferiority, and the neurotic individual draws constantly effective guiding lines for his volition, action and thoughts in the form of traits of character in the broad chaotic field of his soul, in order not to miss the way to the heights, in order to make his security complete. Usually the traits of character tend in a direct line of the masculine ideal in both the male and the female patients, but the neurotic circuitous ways, attacks and predispositions to attack especially following the decisive defeat whose analysis and arrangements in the ensemble reveals the same tendency to the heightening of the masculine ego-consciousness, manifest themselves as in accordance with the above given expositions, even though from an outside view and superficially considered they may appear to be timidity, anxiety, effeminacy, and may be regarded as flight or retreat from the world. The simple question concerning the stability of the far fetched expedient in the form of a neurotic symptom enables us to understand that in these latter cases it is not because a decision has been reached, but because the originally constructed imaginary masculine goal is effective now as it was before and that a cultural adaptation, peace and contentment, cannot be maintained, because the goal is set too high.

Through certain uncertainties of the child concerning his own sex-rôle the masculine element in the guiding fiction is considerably reënforced. In fact one observes that children retain a remarkable interest for differences of sexuality in a hidden form. The similarity of dress in children in the first years, the feminine features in small boys, and masculine in girls, certain threats of the parents as "a boy will change himself into a girl" reproaches to the boy that he is like a girl, to a girl that she is like a boy, may still increase this uncertainty, as long as the differences in the genital organs are unknown. But even where there is the fullest explanation, doubt may awaken through anomalies of the genital organs in erroneous judgments, which may be retained and emerge constantly in later life in the antithetical picture of "masculine-feminine" so that our original statement [10] that the doubt of his own sex-rôle is at the foundation of the neurotic doubt needs extension only in one direction, i.e., that the neurosis holds fast to this condition of doubt

[10] "Psychic Hemaphrodism in Life and in the Neurosis." l. c. and the later publications.

others by one's virtues, to attack others by one's own passivity, to cause pain to others by one's own suffering, to strive to attain the goal of manly force by effeminate means, to make oneself small in order to appear great. Of such sort, however, are often the expedients of neurotics.

Concerning the significance of the most primitive perception and emotion as an abstraction I need waste no words. Just as abstract is the positing of an imaginary guiding point and of this life plan which is now spun out between these two points. With reference to the neurotic psyche we have repeatedly emphasized that it is the greater insecurity which alone tends to withdraw the guiding point still further from reality, to set it higher. In addition to this the inferior sense organs yield qualitatively and quantitatively changed sensations, and the organs of execution a changed technique usually in the sense of greater limitation, so that the self-esteem, the ideal guiding representation, the representation of the world and the life plan must be formed differently from normal representations of this sort, in that they are more abstract, less in conformity with reality. In this process it is true the compensation and over-compensation may sometimes bring the conception of the world and the line of reality nearer together as in the great in the patient subsequently as a security against the necessity of decadency, in order to construct the "hesitating attitude."

The longer the uncertainty as to the sex-rôle exists, the more urgent becomes the effort and tentative preparation to attain the masculine rôle. Thus originates the original picture of the "masculine protest" which has as aim to force the one in whom it exists under all circumstances into the seemingly most masculine attitude, or, as is the case with girls and boys, who early become neurotic, to prevent set-backs in all forms by neurotic expedients, simultaneously, however, to build up directly masculine traits of character and strong affect-predisposition.

The fore-stage of the knowledge of the sex-rôle, that is the period of psychic hermaphroditism of the child exists generally. Attention has been called to its importance by Dessoir and myself. That this stadium with its strong endeavors in the direction of the masculine guiding line is of the greatest significance for the development of the neurosis with its too elevated manly goal and its expedients for gaining security was demonstrated to me by the analysis of the psychoneurosis. Goethe proves himself to be a good observer and connoisseur of nature when he says in Wilhelm Meister's Theatrical Consignment, "Just as at certain periods in their life, children

begin to pay attention to the differences in the sex
of their parents, and their glances through the
envelopes which conceal these secrets bring forth
very wonderful emotions in their nature, so it was
with Wilhelm in this discovery; he was more quiet
and less quiet than before, thought he had learned
something and just from this perceived that he
knew nothing."

In fact one finds as the first expression of this
inexperience and its depressing reaction upon the
psyche an enormous amount of curiosity and
craving for knowledge and in order to find orientation in life notwithstanding this the child comes
under the influence of the guiding line which impels him to act as though he must know everything.   Should he happen to find out the superiority of the manly principle in our society, the
guiding model becomes masculine, especially if
a man, the father appears to him to be the person
with knowledge.

In the case of little girls peculiar traits of character which become especially prominent in the
neurosis develop when they try to hold fast to the
masculine guiding line.   The feeling of having
suffered an injury has just as much weight with
them as for boys who consider themselves female,
so that they put all their interest into collecting
proof of their injury and building up their aggression against their environment.

Imaginary pictures of castration, of man changed to woman, woman to man, of masculine forms of life, emerge in the analysis as indicators of the neurotic psyche, point to the craving for equality with man and permit the masculine fiction to reëmerge constantly in the later changes of form of the guiding line. These neurotics regularly assume an attitude toward life as though they had suffered an injury, or as though they were constantly seeking with the greatest caution, to avoid a loss.

E. H. Meyer says in the "Indo-Germanic Myths" (I. S. 16), "According to the Atharva Veda the Gandharvs (phallic Dæmons) consume the testicles of boys and thus transform the boys into girls." The ideas of many neurotics in childhood seem to have assumed this and similar forms concerning the origination of the two sexes, as if from thoughts concerning a degradation which has been suffered and which assumes the form of a sexual transformation with the woman. The immediate psychical result is then as a rule more acute aggression against the parents, to whom is ascribed the blame for this shortcoming.

Flies, Halban, Weininger, and before them, among others, Schopenhauer and Krafft-Ebing, founded the psychic hermaphroditism on the presence of a hypothetical male and female substance in the individual. Our concept supposes only the antithesis in the valuation of male and female as it actually exists, takes into account the universality of the antithetical figurative apperception-scheme "male-female" and deduces from the pressure of the neurotically reënforced and heightened egotistic ideal the masculine factor which is so easily discoverable. The latter conditions also the emphasis of the feeling of inferiority of the individual by comprehending it in a picture which belongs to the feminine rôle in order to react against it with the character traits, the impulses, and preparations of the masculine protest. The findings published by me have been taken up in a series of the latest works from the Freudian school. A further pursuance of the matter leads irrevocably to a realization of the untenableness of the libido-theory, to a doing away with the sexual etiology and to an understanding of the neurotic sexual conduct as a fiction.

If the masculine protest has thus become clear to us as an expedient of the psyche by means of which it attains full security, and strives to bring itself in conformity with the guiding egotistic idea, it still remains to present to view the formal change of this guiding line as it takes place every time contradictions become apparent in it and the purpose of neurotic efforts to maintain superiority is jeopardized. This is the case when reality threatens the egotistic ideal with degradation. The neurotic in this case will cling more tenaciously to his idea than the normal person. The more deeply, however, he becomes entangled in the reassuring neurosis, the more likely is he, being assisted by memories and warnings, to anticipate an injury, to construct new neurotic circuitous ways, to apply further neurotic expedients for security which for a problem under consideration contain neither a fiat nor a negation, or more likely both at once.

His psychic hermaphroditic character will also manifest itself in the circumstance that he yields, becomes submissive, effeminate, while his efforts at the same time reveal a pressure towards a tendency to dominate, toward manliness, with the result that he makes no progress, because for every step he takes forward he takes one backward, and sometimes even expresses this procedure in pantomime. In the same way the fear of blame, of punishment, of shame, in short of being "down" may alter his straightforward manly traits. The construction of the neurotic feelings of guilt, of congenital criminal instincts, of roughness, of cruelty, and egotism bear fear-inspiring signs in the same ways as the feelings of bashfulness, cowardice, dullness and laziness when these latter are brought neurotically to expression. The bad, intractable child, the years of wild oats, and certain forms of psychoses, frequently the fore-stage of the "developed neurosis," show us the masculine protest in a high, rectilinear development. Their performances are produced directly by the surge of the masculine protest which has become an end in itself and which represents wholly and entirely the reënforced guiding fiction.

Our theoretical presentation of the neurotic psyche would be incomplete, if it did not also enter upon the subject of the nature and significance of dreams. I can in this place advance no well founded theory of dreams, to say nothing of a complete one. But for various reasons I am obliged to communicate all the observations and findings which have rendered possible the study of dreams in the practical part of the work.

Freud's interpretation of dreams was perhaps the greatest step in advance which has been made in our understanding of the psychology of the neuroses. And yet I cannot regard it as the final step in our knowledge of dreams. In the course of an observation of dreams extending over many years of healthy and unhealthy persons I have arrived at the following result:

1. The dream is a sketch-like reflection of psychic attitudes and indicates for the investigator the characteristic manner in which the dreamer takes his attitude in regard to a certain problem.

It coincides therefore, with the form of the fictitious guiding line, yields only efforts of premeditation, tentative preparations of an aggressive attitude and can therefore be utilized to great advantage for the purpose of understanding these individual preparations, predispositions, and the guiding fiction itself.

2. In the same way there comes to light in the dream, in a more or less abstract manner, the dreamer's attitude towards the world about him as well as his traits of character [11] and their neurotic abnormalities. The abstraction in dream-thought is necessitated by the craving for security, which seeks to solve a problem by simplifying it and by referring it to a less complete infantile stage. This it accomplishes in a manner which is true of thinking generally, except that it is more profound. It makes use too of memory, and in a figurative analogical manner, through the hallucinatory awakening of memories of a fear-inspiring or energy-exciting sort. The exclusion of reality by sleep favors the abstract thinking in dreams, as correction is to a great part prevented by the insensibility of the sense organs. To this circumstance as well as to the absence of a conscious positing of purpose in

[11] G. Chr. Lichtenberg already wrote—If people were to relate accurately their dreams, their character cou'd be read from them sooner than from the face.

dream thought is due the incomprehensibility of the contents of dreams, which only receive meaning when taken as symbols of life, as an "as if" for which the interpretation has to supply the real aggression.

3. These facts which still remain to be proved as well as the form of expression of the dream in an "as if" ("It seemed to me as if") reveal to us the nature of the dream as a factor in which those tentative efforts and tasks become manifest by which caution seeks to gain the mastery of a situation in the future. In the dreams of neurotic persons it is possible, therefore, to observe more distinctly than in others the neurotic methods of apperception which work according to the principle of an antithesis, the emphasized feeling of inferiority and the guiding egotistic idea, or to divine them in connection with the mental life of these persons.

4. The tendency of the neurotically reënforced guiding idea will be revealed regularly in the dreams of a neurotic person, usually in the form of a striving to attain a position "above" or the masculine protest. The feminine or "under" base of operation is always indicated.

5. Repeated dreams of the same content and dreams of childhood reveal the fictitious guiding line most distinctly. Because they construct themselves upon a completed scheme or one that

is in a condition to be used which is erected and sustained by the neurotic final purpose. The various dreams of a night indicate this attempt at various solutions and are a characteristic of the feeling of extreme uncertainty. The so-called censor of dreams by means of which is accomplished a concealment or disguising of actual facts by distortion, reveals itself as the craving for security which accomplishes the formal change of the fiction in the neurosis as well as in the dream, and seeks to avoid by a circuitous way a contradiction in the masculine guiding line. Other disfigurations are inherent in the nature of the more abstract dream thinking and in its character as a mere reflection.

6. The symbolisms and expedients of analogy in dreams are radiations containing forms and contents of dynamic affect reënforcements, their word-pictures, so to speak. They are a psychic superstructure over a compromise between a psychic situation and a biased, usually falsified, sophistically applied souvenir which must supply the resonance required by the idea.

The fulfillment of infantile wishes in dreams asserted by Freud is solved by me by regarding it as the effect of premeditation to attain security, whereby memories grouped together with a view to a certain effect are taken as helps in the form of mementoes, a psychic expedient which also dominates all logical thinking, and which are not the libidinous or sexual wishes of childhood.

The only difference between the neurosis and normality with its dreams and its delusions is the heightened tendency brought about by the reenforced fiction, to choose those memories which have been made effective, in short the neurotic perspective,—the neurotic does not suffer from reminiscences, he makes them.

If this point of comparison, an absolutely necessary one for orientation and certainty in action, becomes once fixed, a point which is in proportion to the degree with which the feeling of inferiority weighs upon the child, this point must for the above given reasons, from the necessity of making comparisons, and on account of the adjustments which take place in childhood, become stable, hypostasized and regarded as holy, as divine. On the one hand are the real conditions and activities of the subject; on the other hand are the compensatory result of the feeling of inferiority, the Deity, the guiding idea apperceived in the form of a person or an event. This latter ideal point operates now as though all directing forces were contained in it. Thus first arises from an organic, objective life that which we call soul life, the psyche.

Every step the child takes directs itself according to this system and is in turn directed by it.

There is a continuous weighing, feeling, preparation, formation of predispositions and measuring on the ideal which brings the child forward in his development. He measures himself with men as well as with women, whereby the contrast between the sexes furnishes a guide and produces a psychic adjustment in accordance with a contrast in a certain sense in a hostile, evasive direction in the masculine line. In the neurotically disposed child, the compensatory craving for security heightened by the feeling of uncertainty is responsible, through the over-stimulation of attention in this direction for the abstract, neurotically reënforced directing lines to the high-flown goal of the masculine protest. And the more sharply defined understanding of the contrast of the sexes produces earlier and more profoundly the preparatory attitudes toward the opposite sex, the more so when, as is the case with neurotics, the exclusively masculine appraisal of the ideal reflects upon his feeling of inferiority causing it to appear feminine.

The nature of home training carries with it the result that in his first attempts at formulating an ideal of personality, the child pictures to himself traits belonging to the most important member of the family, usually the father. Neurotically disposed children who in contrasting themselves with the father experience an accentuation of their feeling of inferiority, immediately hit upon preparatory expedients and construct devices for combat as though they were obliged to demonstrate their superiority to the father. In these preparatory efforts is contained also the attitude to the opposite sex, in so far as the intellect of the child does not make a mistake in regard to his own sexual rôle, and many of his predispositions which are to come into effectiveness later in life are tentatively practiced in a playful manner upon members of the family of the opposite sex, in the waking state or in hallucinations, or in his dreams.

That along with this the mother serves in a certain sense as a model for the boy has long been known and has been mentioned by Nietzsche. The boundary itself which the child sets for himself is also a matter of experiment for him. His wishes are, if he be neurotically disposed, boundless. Discontented because of the too great distance to his egotistic ideal, he even goes so far as to entertain sexual wishes in regard to the mother, a proof of how boundless is the "will to power." A fixation of a sexual relation, however, must have other grounds than chance wishes in the field of boundless aspirations. The desire of the boy extends to other female persons with whom he is brought into contact. The picture if then again similar to that of possession "to wish to possess the mother" becomes a sign of his discontent, a symbol of his boundless aspirations, of his obstinacy and his fear of other women. Now in later life a "fixation" on the mother from similar constellations may result, not however, because the wish was heretofore libidinous. For it is a matter of indifference of what nature the real relation to the mother was—the psyche of the neurotic will always utilize it in some way for the purpose of furnishing him security.

The motive of the discontent interests us here above all. It originates from the feeling of having suffered an injury and it is obvious that the child waits fulfillment of every aspiration in his "growing up." According to the psychology of the "as if" he may expect his cure from the development of his hair, his teeth, his genital organs. His experience with his teeth serves to give him the impression that a thing may grow again. The tooth-motive plays a frequent rôle in the dreams and phantasies with girls in order to enable them to cling to their hope of becoming a man, with boys to give hope to their longing for a more complete manhood. If a tooth is pulled, a milk tooth, a new, stronger one forms. The pulling out of teeth, therefore, symbolizes in the dream the wish to become a man.

Neurotic men like women are full of the feeling of having suffered an injury and their whole life

is spent in the effort at enlarging their spheres of
influence. In order to attain this, indeed, in
order even to assume their attitude toward this
effort, they are obliged to keep up constantly
their discontent, so that they will find nourish-
ment for it and proof of their neglect in every situation by examining it, rearranging it or arbitrarily changing it, but always keeping in mind the
fictitious guiding goal. With great regularity,
I found in them the apperception according to the
antithetical scheme "male-female" by means of
which they sought and classified all their experiences. This scheme according to which they wish
to arrange the cosmic picture is usually overlayed
by an antithetical picture of the large and small
masculine genitalia. It is a frequent and characteristic discovery that a finer sensibility develops at points of the body which by nature are
inferior, whose excitability sometimes takes the
character of pleasurable sensations. I have described this phenomenon in the "Studie uber Or-
ganmin derwertigheit" (1907, Wien und Berlin)
and refer them to the compensatory adjustment
which has come into play during the individual's
experience in his struggle for existence where the
organs or parts of organs in question were menaced. These compensatory, now higher valued
portions of an inferior organ—inferior after they
had suffered an injury in their ascendancy—are

really in a certain sense protective adjustments, although frequently they do not prove of worth. Because, however, their technique has become different and no longer keeps pace with the nearly normal organ, the psychic phenomena connected with these organs are striking and deviate from normality. This is the same albeit more minute variation based upon somatic inferiority of which I have spoken in the biology, i.e., explanation of variation, refinement and decline of an organ.[12]

In this way, for instance, the sense of taste has evolved as a security-serving apparatus, in the realm of the nutritive organ, but along with this also the pleasure sense apparatus which must now guarantee the continuance of nutrition as well as the proper choice of food.

The variation from the type is brought about by the "compensation tendency" which is already introduced in the germ plasm.

The environment (in a broader sense the milieu) dominates the "germ plasm" and in this manner is explained the prompt uniformity of reaction, viz. "inferiority plus compensatory se-

[12] Thus the "value of an organ" likewise becomes a symbol in life's current in which are reflected the past, present, future as well as the fictive goal in like manner as is the case with the individual's make-up or with the neurotic symptoms. The idea of the "symbolic in a person's appearance" is not a new one. It has been expressed by Porta, Gall and Carus.

curity," through a change in the conditions of life in the broadest sense, that is to say, all particular members of a single species vary in the same way when the same change in their mode of life takes place. In regard to human society one must keep constantly in mind, more so than in the animal and vegetable kingdoms—that the demands on the single individual vary to a considerable degree one from the other, both quantitatively and qualitatively, so that their somatic inferiorities and the compensatory adjustments resulting therefrom differ very widely. And their variations would be still more striking were it not for the fact that the human psyche has thrust itself into the circle of correlations and compensations with such preponderance as the principal organ of adjustive security.[13] Now the standard tendencies to security are no longer variations in the organs themselves, but psychic peculiarities. There always continues to exist a connection

[13] The psychic adjustment of man with its preparations and peculiar characteristics simulates so very closely the adjustive variations in the animal sphere, that children, neurotics, poets and even speech itself utilize this analogy for the purpose of elucidating by way of comparison a psychic gesture, a trait of character, a type of preparedness by means of a representation of an animal, as is the case for instance in the designing of escutcheons, in poetic similes, in fables and parable. See also Erckmann's Chatrain, the famous Dr. Malthieu, Goethe's Reinecke Fox, painting and caricatures.

which can be sufficiently proved, and we are able to infer from somatic variations stigmata and signs of degeneration of the same, that there has taken place an increased compensatory adjustment of the brain and more acentuated tendencies to obtain security. The nature and tendency of all psychic processes are full of the efforts of precaution and defensive preparations for gaining superiority so that one cannot avoid the conclusion that what we term soul, spirit, reason and understanding are for us abstractions of those effective guiding lines, to which human beings reach out beyond the sphere of bodily sensations, striving to overstep their limitations in order to gain the mastery of a portion of the world and to secure themselves against threatened dangers. The imperfection of the independently acting organ is thus magically elevated to that security which is furnished by knowledge, understanding and foresight.

In the animal kingdom the function performed in men by the understanding is performed by a finely adjusted technical apparatus. The fine scent of the dog becomes superfluous or is brought under man's service, the highly specialized sense of taste, which teaches cattle to avoid poisonous plants, is supplied in man by the understanding eye.

But it is the same tendency which continues through eternity the struggle of the ancestors to facilitate the preservation of life by more finely graded, sharply differentiated organs as well as by more refined expedients of the psyche.

And thus it is permitted to us, to regard this sort of more sensitive peripheral apparatus, its special physiognomy and mimic as a sign of an imperfection of some organ, as a trace which betrays a transmitted somatic defect. This is also true of the extraordinary development of the organs of taste in man, for the greater sensibility to stimuli of the lips and mucous membrane of the mouth, with which there is usually associated a more exacting state of the gums, alimentary canal, and stomach.

Physiognomically the picture of the more inferior mouth is represented in the form of more mobile, thicker or thinner lips, usually associated with slight deformities of the lips, of the tongue (lingua scrotallis Schmidt), of the gums, with which are often associated signs of degeneration of these parts, enlarged tonsils or of the whole status lymphaticus. At times, it is true, all higher development in the sense of a tendency to compensation is wanting in the presence of an inferiority, even the hyperasthesia. Reflex anomalies are quite common, sometimes exaggeration, sometimes diminution of the pharyngeal reflex; along with defects of childhood, one observes a greater occupation with the mouth, as touching of the mouth, thumb sucking, tendencies to put everything into the mouth, vomiting. Along with this, good digestion is usually present in so far as this is not prevented by other coexisting somatic defects.

But the evil, the deprivation and the pain which from the cradle on are the fate of the child with an inferior alimentary tract, awake in him at the same time a feeling of inferiority, of having suffered an injury and of uncertainty and force the constitutionally predisposed child to a resort to fictive expedients. The over-strongly developed, precocious, egotistic ideal includes within itself also fictitious goals of over-gratifications which reality can never satisfy. The attention of such children is directed after the manner of a compulsory idea to all problems of nutrition and their sublimation (Nietzsche). The deprivation of a delicacy releases in them entirely different emotions and actions than we would expect. Their sense turns to the kitchen, their play and the infantile choice of vocation turn on the phantasy of procuring nutrition, to be cook or candymaker. The importance of money as a means to power dawns upon them earlier and more forcibly, as well as the sense of greed and economy. Stereotypies and pedantries in eating are often revealed, courses of action according to a principle such as the best is to be put into the mouth first or last, the impatient preferring the first practice, the cautious and avaricious the latter. Idiosyncrasies against certain foods, refusal of food, hasty swallowing, are often adhered to as traits of obstinacy and show the application of the problem of nutrition as an aggression against the parents. Aside from the organic diseases of later life which go with an inferior alimentary apparatus, and among which I have emphasized ulcer of the stomach, appendicitis, cancer, diabetes, liver and gall bladder disease, there is manifested in the neurosis a stronger participation and frequent employment of functional disturbances of the digestive tract. Its intimate relation to the psyche is reflected in many neurotic and psychotic symptoms. I believe I am on the track of a special expedient of this sort, without being able to present conclusive facts. A number of neurotic symptoms, such as erythrophobia, neurotic obstipation and colic, asthma, probably also vertigo, vomiting, headache, and migraine stand in some sort of relation, which is as yet not entirely clear to me, with a voluntary but unconsciously coöperating activity of anus-contraction ("cramp" of the other authors) (spasms of sigmoid flexure, Holzknecht, Singer) and that of abdominal pressure, symbolic acts which are ac-

complished through the domination of the reënforced fiction.

Acquisitiveness and greed for gold and power
I found strikingly in the foreground and as essential factors in the egotistic ideal of these individuals.

PRACTICAL PART

CHAPTER I

AVARICE, SUSPICIOUSNESS, ENVY, CRUELTY, THE
    DEROGATORY CRITIQUE OF THE NEUROTIC,
    NEUROTIC APPERCEPTION, SENILE NEUROSES,
    CHANGES IN THE FORM AND INTENSITY OF
    THE FICTION. SOMATIC JARGON (ORGAN-
    JARGON)

I WISH to speak first of those traits of character which may be demonstrated with a certain
regularity in all neurotics, and which reach expression in the patient's striving with great
eagerness, directly or circuitously, consciously or
unconsciously, by means of purposive thinking
and acting, or through an especial arrangement
of symptoms, towards greater possession, towards a heightening of his power and influence,
towards a degradation and belittling of others.
All these forms of self-interest are most often
found to coexist, and it is only after a better
insight that one recognizes the mighty preponderance of those evasions by means of which the
patient deceives himself and his environment.
He even deceives also science.

While playing, for instance, the rôle of unselfishness, one finds again and again in his attacks, in his neurosis, moreover in the end result gained by means of the latter, that exaggerated eagerness of which we have spoken in the beginning:—He thus arouses the impression of a double-ego, of one suffering from a splitting of consciousness, and whereas a fictitious goal permits him to observe secretly more rigidly than does the normal person the scheme of avarice, envy, desire for mastery, malice, disputatiousness, and desire to please (coquetry), he is compelled in the open (perhaps also on account of his desire to please) to play the rôle of the benefactor and patron, of the pacifier and unselfish saint. Not that this play is usually without disastrous results, somewhat like Gregor Werles' truth—fanaticism in Ibsen's "Wild Duck." One cannot estimate strongly enough the neurotic's mania to desire possession of everything, his eagerness to wish to be the first one—cannot be over-stated—even though the obvious traits of character furnish the most contradictory picture. What really drives the patient onward is the overweening desire for absolute power; and inasmuch as his ego-consciousness takes offense at many of his means—inasmuch as the power of others may prevent his triumph, he conceals the hindering traits of character from himself and others, and having full insight into his hostile impulses and their unpopularity, he allows himself to be guided in the open in his conscious activities by the ideal of virtue. Notwithstanding this, however, his heightened aggressive tendency betrays itself—namely in the dreams in uncontrolled acts, in his attitude, mimicry and gesture—and in that psychic being ("Geschehen") the expression for which is the neurosis.

Concerning the question of transmissibility of such characteristics, yes, also their antagonistic arrangement, there as a rule develops that they have been acquired as secondary guiding principles after the pattern of the father, the mother, or representative persons and are in nowise inherited. The neurotic psyche finds it in its own or in some representative material, for the purpose of which the "double play"—the cleft consciousness of society—is utilized in many cases. It is then, however, the device of the neurosis, to conceal and change those hostile aggressive traits which are frequently unsuitable for the fictitious purpose of obtaining a heightening of the ego-consciousness—and to obtain the latter goal through a more intensive utilization of artifices— often by means of contrasting characteristics and neurotic symptoms. One readily becomes convinced that the generosity of such patients obeys the same goal of the "will to power" which the patient strives to approach also through the heightening of his aggressive tendency, his avarice and thriftiness.

One of my patients who came under my observation on account of stammering and depressive states, permitted to appear in his environment a detection only of his generosity. One day he made a voluntary bequest to a certain institute, and told me this story with an apparently directly associated statement that he felt unusually depressed that day. Along with this his stammering likewise became more pronounced. The exaggerated state of his neurosis showed itself to be a result of his generosity as result of which he feels himself degraded and one is justified in expecting a revelation of the real working of this individual in further acts, thoughts and dreams as running with the developing neurotic symptoms—not because he has repressed his avariciousness or a corresponding sexual impulse—but because he has deviated too far from his goal— namely, to increase his possessions. He must therefore do something which will bring him back to it. He tells me further, "It was already far after the dinner hour. I felt very hungry, and besides a friend awaited me in a restaurant where we were to dine together. I had to walk therefore the (long) distance to that place. My friend still waited. After dinner I felt somewhat better." This means that he began at once to save again and made the journey on foot, notwithstanding hunger, depression and rendezvous. Incidentally, he was able to let the friend wait, which is with many neurotics the concealed mode of asserting their desire for dominancy.

The very first manifestation, actions and communications of the patient in the presence of the physician, frequently contain the most important of the disease mechanism and character development.   This is so because the patient is as yet not in possession of cautiousness in the presence of the physician.   As the above quoted patient introduced himself to me, he told me casually, that his father was not well to do, and that he was unable to make great sacrifices for the treatment. After a certain time, there came of necessity to light that he deceived me in this respect in order to obtain a smaller charge.   He showed himself to be avaricious also in many other respects, but at the same time he endeavored to deceive both himself and others in this respect.   Both of these traits were also possessed by the father, and our patie..t was taught stinginess by the latter with special stress.   He was often told "money is might, for money everything can be had."   Thus it could not be avoided that our patient, who was already in childhood very ambitious and tyrannical, having later fallen into an uncertain situation and believing that he could not reach the paternal standard, through direct means, took refuge under the pressure of his ambitiousness, in the device to convince the father of his utter helplessness and of the other failures of his educational plans, by retaining this childhood defect, stammering. Through his stammering, he spoiled his father's play—because he was not able to be the first one, because he was not able to surpass the latter.

Our culture, however, agrees with those children who see in the amassing of fortune the road to power. Similarly led on, this "will to power" assumed the external form of stinginess and avarice in so far as he further developed these tendencies. It was only the contradiction between a vulgar avariciousness and the ego-ideal which forced him to a concealment of the impulse to avarice by means of which he wished to dominate his father, and forced him to the substitution of the stammering. In the further course of the analysis the origin of his desire for possession became evident. He suffered practically constantly in his infancy from stomach and intestinal disorders, which were the expression of a hereditary inferiority of the gastro-intestinal tract. In the family, stomach and intestinal disorders played an important rôle. The patient recalled very distinctly how he frequently had to deny himself appetizing food in spite of hunger and desire, whereas his parents and brothers and sisters consumed them with pleasure. Whenever he could he gathered foods, bonbons and fruits to be feasted upon later. In this tendency to gather, we already see the influence of the developing craving for security, which is constantly endeavoring to adjust in some way or other the feeling of degradation.

How far, however, this may reach may be shown by a constructed example which I am able to verify with analogies from our case. The eagerness for power, and through it for possession may be stirred up by the feeling of inferiority to such a point that one finds it at phases of the psychic development when one would least expect it.

A small patient of this sort will at first, it is true, only desire to have the apple which is forbidden him, in seeing his father and brother eating the same. Envy will begin to stir itself, and after a brief period such a child may have reached the stage in his deliberateness and contemplation when out of the striving for equality he will attempt to prevent others from having anything before he has it. It will soon have reached so far in the elaboration of this albeit only slightly important idea, as to have at his disposal all sorts of preparations and facilities, it will, especially in the presence of an originally inferior muscular system, train itself for the whole year by climbing and jumping in order to be able to climb a tree as a master in the fall.   The human psyche is not able to account always for fictitious goals, and thus the child may apparently free himself from his goal, employ his dexterity in sports and gymnastics in the service of other tendencies, which serve in a different manner his ego-consciousness somewhat like our modern States conduct our war preparations without even knowing the future enemy.

The father of our patient may have easily been taken by the boy as an incidental example because he excelled his environment in greatness, power, wealth and social standing.   If the boy is to emerge out of his insecurity into which he has been plunged by his constitutional inferiority he must arrange his preparations for life in accordance with a set point of view as after a plan (blue print).   A marked exhibition of the guiding principle toward the paternal ideal (Vaterideal) is in itself quite a neurotic trait, because in it we may comprehend the entire misery of the child who endeavors to emerge from his insecurity. The craving for security (Sicherungstendenz) of the neurosis leads the patient in this way out of the sphere of his own power and forces him into a path which leads away from reality, first because he takes for his object his fiction to be equal to his father or even to excel him and is therefore forced to formulate, arrange and influence his apperception of life under its compulsion, and second because one can never succeed in carrying out such a fiction in real life except in a psychosis.

In this way, there develops in the psyche of the child an intensive searching, weighing, and measuring tendency of which I shall have to say something more. That which is according to my experience primarily responsible for the too rigid assumption of the paternal guiding principles, may be discovered in an investigation into the sexual rôles. The neurotically predisposed child, or as I may say, the child laboring under the pressure of a feeling of inferiority, desires to become a man, as soon as the neurosis develops, to be a man. In both instances he can only conduct himself in such a manner as if he were a man or shall become one. The exaggerated craving for security drives also in this instance the attitude of the developing neurotic into the ban of the fiction, so that in some instances even conscious simulation may come into play, and a girl for instance in order to escape a feeling of inferiority may in the beginning borrow in conscious imitation masculine gestures of her father. There is no reason for the assumption that because of this she must be in love with her father. The mere overvaluation of the masculine principle suffices for this, may nevertheless at times be taken as infatuation by the girl herself as well as by her environment, should the preparations for the future playfully demand a hinting of love or a marriage. In our case the guiding line to the compensatory ego-ideal, transformed itself through a change of form and content into a craving to excel the father in wealth, esteem, and along with this in manliness.   The inquiry into his own sexual rôle, sets in intensively and typically as sexual curiosity, whereby the patient in his feeling of inferiority, apperceives the smallness of his infantile genitals as compared with the largeness of the paternal ones, as a bitter setback, as a want of masculinity.   His ambitiousness which shall enable him to rise out of his state of inferiority, compelled him to a heightening of his sense of shame, in order that his genitals may not be seen in the event of an exposure (in case he is nude). To this may be added that he was of Jewish descent.   He had heard certain things about circumcision and harbored the idea that he was also (Verkürzt) belittled through the operation. His masculine protest drove him to a degradation of woman, as if he had to give proof to his superiority in this wise, and came into the most abominable relationship with his mother.

But also with respect to his father, whose preference for himself he gained through diplomatic adjustment, he harbored hostile thoughts which became especially prominent when the father over-emphasized his own superiority to do which he had a marked inclination. In this chaos of feelings the patient sought orientation, and found it only in the thought to become superior to his father, to become more manly than he.

He had, too, as often happens in such cases, undertaken attempts at enlarging his genitals or bringing about erection. This route which leads to sexual precocity and masturbation, was soon abandoned by him, because his father warned him against it on numerous occasions. Thus there remained as a substitution for his masculine protest, only efforts to become richer, more honored and wiser than his father, and to degrade his environment.

His father placed great hopes in the patient's oratorical talents, which had shown themselves already in childhood, did not allow himself to be deceived by the mild stammering of the boy, and hoped he would make a law career. In this respect the patient was able to strike at the father's most vulnerable point, and thus he sank into a more pronounced stammering, a neurotic manifestation of the insurance against the superiority of the father, a manifestation whose inception was given him by a stammering home teacher.

In the course of time, this symptom gained many other uses, for example, the one that through his stammering he always gained time in which to weigh his words, to avoid demands of the family, to utilize the confession of others as well as that prejudice because of which, only little was expected of him, which he then managed to fulfill easily.   It is interesting that his quite apparent stammering was no obstacle to his courtship, that it even expedited matters, a fact which becomes quite comprehensible from our standpoint, according to which we assume the existence of a quite prevalent type of girl which cannot omit from the conditions of their love that the man of their choice must be beneath them, so that they may with certainty rule over him.   Especially hostile feelings against his parents, brothers and sisters and the servants he put a stop to, through the development of a new guiding principle which was to make of him a benevolent man.   This new evolution took place under a nightly confession through which he reproached himself for his wickedness and arranged qualms of conscience.   His growing knowledge thus showed him the way, through a cultural subterfuge to a heightening of his ego-consciousness.

The want of a direct aggressiveness showed itself in thoughts and phantasies, albeit also in his good progress at school, so that he was victorious

over all his classmates.   A growing tendency towards sarcasm and exasperation of others was at
this time the only manifest expression of his former often violent aggressiveness which gained for
him the nickname of "blood-leech."   His combative attitude played an important rôle in the cause
of Judaism, which was reflected in an act of compulsion at the age of twelve.   Whenever he entered a swimming pool he had to cover his genitals with his hands and immediately submerge his
head under the water, where he kept it until he
counted 49, so that he often came to the surface
gasping for air and exhausted.   The analysis revealed the mental content to be a striving of his
phantasy to bring about an equality of genitalia.
The forty-ninth year is, according to the old Jewish laws, with which he had become acquainted
shortly before, the year of the jubilee, in which
all acres were again made equal.   Ideas of this
sort, and the simultaneous concealment of the
genitalia showed the way to the interpretation.
One may almost draw the conclusion that also his
stammering was intended to make him quits with
a superiority of his father, of all people, inasmuch
as his stuttering was an obstacle to them, was even
painful to them.

His avarice, his stinginess, were accordingly
active in the same direction, namely, to clear the
field of superiorities of others, to insure him

against further degradation and belittling through poverty, thus he was compelled markedly to expand these secondary directions and to formulate and evaluate his experiences according to them in order to reach the heightening of his ego-consciousness, his masculine protest. It was only under such circumstances where through revelation of these traits of character a lowering of his ego might arise that he suppressed their apparent activity.

It were an absurdity to wish to assume a moral standpoint in a medico-psychological question, to consider people like the above as morally inferior. Those who have an inclination in this direction I wish to remind of the very strong, compensatory traits of character, of a worthy nature, for the rest I wish to remind them of Rochefoucauld's wise sentence—viz: "I have never investigated the soul of a wicked man, but I once became acquainted with the soul of a good man: I was shocked."

In another case, the nature of the avarice showed itself not as a safety device for the compensation of a feeling of degradation, but above all as an artifice in the service of the craving for security. A forty-five year old patient who suffered throughout life from psychic impotency, and was pursued by suicidal ideas, showed an especially marked tendency to degrade others.

We know this trait of character from the description of the previous case where it served as it always does to do away with one's own feeling of inferiority. With this tendency there is usually associated exaggerated mistrust and envy, which have for their object as neurotic-psychic dexterities, the falsification of the search and valuation of experiences. A tendency, too, to cause others bodily and psychic pain, will likewise know how to assert itself in an accentuated manner. The abstract, guiding point of view of the patient, to assure his dominating position, to be above, appeared to be obviously threatened, and compelled a strengthening of fictitious guiding principles. Reminiscences out of his infantile period were utilized in the neurosis, as result of which he came near being the victim of a homosexualist. He was raised as an only boy among his sisters, a situation which, according to my experience, frequently narrows the understanding of one's own sexual rôle.

Of importance was his attitude toward his father, because it likewise drove him to strengthened security devices. The father, namely, was brutal, egotistical, tyrannical, so that it was difficult for the boy to assert his own value in his presence. Several love adventures had thrown the father into quite difficult situations which our patient utilized as mementoes in his developed psychosis. This mistrust was directed against all women. Throughout life he remained ready to make sacrifices for his sisters, but he had already apperceived this fact with an unusual amount of feeling, and readily developed from this trains of thought which were to show how readily he gave in to women. Incidentally, he was able to advance quite considerably in this direction in order to be able to emphasize sharply this impression for himself. It was then that he was prepared to withdraw himself from women.

He transformed into a sexual image, feelings of inferiority which were present in his childhood. The reason for his unmanly bearing—for the homosexualist wanted to take him for a girl—he sought for and found in an incidental Cryptorchism caused by a patent canal. At the age of eight he watched a boy in the act of masturbation. *Hic puer ei semen ejacularit in os*—which he looked upon as a further sign of his feminine rôle. So long as he took his father as his guiding principle, he exhibited the ordinary dexterities intended to make him equal to his father. He secretly consumed his father's whiskey, endeavored to bring his mother over to his side, and already early in life had chosen his father's trade, by means of which he was also able to satisfy his sadistic tendencies which were excited by his feeling of inferiority and his striving toward the paternal guiding line—to choose the trade of a butcher. He was also fond of bringing his vulgar tendencies into execution upon girls and women—he was in the habit of biting them, beating them, and took part one time in a sexual assault, when he carried out *coitus per anum* in order to avoid a possibility of alimony. His experience, however, which showed him in the complete brutal character of his father, drove him, because of the threatening of a lawsuit, and the degradation associated with it, to a neurotic subterfuge. He utilized his already accentuated mistrust of women for the purpose of torturing them with fits of jealousy, of bringing them entirely under his influence and insure in this manner the appearance of dominancy.

His *ejaculatio præcox* and the associated impotency served his need for security in the same manner as did his animosity towards women. He showed preference for the seduction of married women in order to cause them disappointments through his impotency, at the same time, however, to gain in a sportive manner a substantiation of his belief that all women were bad. Also in his compulsory ideas this tendency to cause pain manifested itself. Thus even during his treatment he experienced sudden impulsions to bite and beat a language teacher while taking a lesson from her, because he developed ideas that she had a lover whom she preferred to the patient. This sadistic reaction to a feeling of subordinacy, as a masculine protest against a feeling of being unmanly, effeminate, had its origin in childhood and runs through his entire neurosis. It was not difficult to prove, that his impotency similarly obeyed the goal to find a means whereby to escape the call of love, the subordination to a wife, a tendency, however, which found its continuation in a further degradation of women.

As he saw no prospect of dominating his teacher, he immediately left her, because he knew that she was dependent upon giving him lessons. Before, however, having done this he undertook a critical estimation of the expense of taking lessons, found them beyond his means which could be readily seen to be a false purposive valuation of the very well-to-do individual. In the same manner he made use of the occasionally recurring reminiscences of incestuous thoughts, in order to become apprehensively conscious of his inferiority, of his criminal tendencies as soon as women came into play. Thus he established his base of operation, by means of which he must insure himself against the feminine gender, as a result of which he seemed to be assured of lasting superiority throughout life.

The essence of his compulsion towards an insurance against women lay in the fear that he

might experience in marriage or love disappointment which he might attribute to his unmanliness.   Inasmuch as he sought his remote goal in
the proof of his might he was bound to become
inclined toward caution and neurotic subterfuges.   In this patient also there were present
early gastro-intestinal disturbances, and as a
peripheral sign of inferiority the fatal inguinal
hernia.   In his sort of love-activity, exaggerated
avarice lent itself as the most useful means for
an insurance against a too far-reaching surrender.   In order, however, that this avarice may be
of use, it must embrace the whole sphere of his
life's relations and must be omnipresent.   It
must in turn be supported, it must be assisted by
all sorts of by-traits.   This took place among
other things in the arrangement of compulsory
ideas.   Whenever he used an automobile, the
thought that a collision might take place came to
his mind.   A further analysis of this compulsory
idea revealed that he was farthest away from a
belief in such an eventuality but that he always
avoided all expensive means of travel.   Yes,
even when he used the tram cars for an extended
trip, the thought occurred to him, upon reaching the point where the cheap fare terminated
and the more expensive one began, that a collision might take place, or that the bridge which
had to be crossed might collapse, so that he would

always pay the cheaper fare, save a few pennies
and cover the rest of the distance on foot. He
was on the road where he felt bitterly every expenditure.

Thus it also came to pass that he sought to
degrade man, in order to gain a uniformity of
behavior. This already became distinctly manifest in the hunt after married women, and the
dismay and disappointment of the seduced women
as well as the abusive language which he used toward them afterward pleased him no less than
the satisfaction of once again having shown himself to be the stronger. This was in line with
the content of his life, with the change of form
in which his original fiction to be the manliest
came closest to realization.

Only the fear of women which synchronously
with the realization of his own femininity originally led him to his exaggerated masculine protest, found itself again in the unduly accentuated insurance against the domination of women
and allowed him to strengthen beyond measure
like a safety-dam his mistrust and avarice, both
of which offered good arguments. Swept away
by this craving for security, he furthermore attached to it his psychic impotency, with which he
became acquainted during his first attempts at
coitus. A servant girl whom he wanted to se-
duce as a youngster, offered resistance and es-

caped him by tightening her limbs.   He was at that time inexperienced and considered himself impotent.   Later, as he became more experienced in these matters, he felt his inexperience in such a way, as if woman were an insoluble puzzle to him.   In the original impotency, however, as well as in his helplessness in the presence of woman, he found the neurotic subterfuges by means of which to escape a depreciatory defeat, a decision adverse to his masculinity.   The comparing of himself with other men set in vehemently now.   He would surprise himself for instance, when sitting at the table in company, in a psychic situation, where before any one even had spoken a word, he was already planning a repartee, already figuring how he might prove the speaker wrong, no matter whether he was speaking of a book or a theatrical performance, or society or place, his derogatory criticism always pushed itself to the front in a most pronounced form.   And so it was to be expected that after a brief introductory period his traits of mistrust, avarice, and depreciation of others would become evident every time he underwent medical treatment, often quite artfully linked one with the other.   This phenomenon, not at all in the Freudian sense of a transference, but because his rigidly fixed psychic gesture, his attitude of attack, his tendency to degrade others, actually did, and upon closer acquaintance, was obliged to come to the surface.   To this was added another accentuating moment.   His object when seeking the advice of a physician, could not have been simply to become rid of his impotency because in such an event, he would have been cast into the chaos of his apprehensions.   He was much more anxious to find proof of his incurability, or to find means of ridding himself of his impotency without the fear of a defeat.   In order to bring about the first, a depreciation of the physician's ability was a preliminary condition.   The proper means of ridding himself of his impotency however, he could only find after following up his fear of women to its source, to the feeling of his unmanliness, in which his feeling of inferiority became concrete.   One of his dreams which occurred at the period preceding the termination of the treatment showed this state of affairs very distinctly.

I must first of all briefly state that I make use of certain important parts of the Breuer-Freud technique of dream interpretation, but that I see in the dream an abstracting, simplifying endeavor to find, by means of a premeditation and testing of difficulties carried on in accordance with the patient's own peculiar scheme—a protective way for the ego-consciousness out of a situation which threatens a defeat.

One will therefore always discover in the

dream, that significant scheme of the antithetical
mode of apperception: "masculine-feminine,"
"above—beneath" as existing originally in everybody, but especially marked in the neurotic.
The various notions and recollections which come
to the surface in the dream, must be brought
within this scheme before they can be of any aid
in the interpretation of same, whose object it is
not—or at least not principally—the fulfillment
of infantile wishes but rather to accompany those
introductory endeavors, to bring about a balance
in favor of the ego-consciousness, through balancing the patient's debit-credit account in a peculiarly neurotic manner.   His dream was as follows:

"I dealt in second-hand goods in Vienna, or in
Germany, or in France. I had to buy, however,
new goods and wash them, because this would
then be cheaper. Then they were again old
(second-hand) goods."

The new goods meant new potent genitalia in
contrast to the "(second-hand) old goods," his
impotency—which as yet nobody had cured.
Here the idea of a new life, of a possibility of attaining potency, shines through. The words,
"because they would be cheaper" correspond to
the previously elucidated ideas, his fear of money
expenditures in case he does not become potent.
This idea, however, can only be accepted under

one condition, to wit—if the patient is saturated with the conviction that he is boundless in his love-impulse, that he knows no limits and senselessly hunts after women. This conviction he purposely takes for himself out of his childhood reminiscences, out of his period of puberty and adolescence. In doing so he also assists in the shaping of his infantile incest-stirrings should these serve his purpose in a form, as if he had coveted his mother or sisters with a sexual object. This means that he works, with a fiction which arose from the assumed goal, through gaining security for himself, similarly as Sophocles developed and shaped the Œdipus legend in order to stabilize the holy commands of the gods. Our patient became a willing victim of his limited understanding of dialectic and of the antithetical manner of primitive thinking. The guiding idea of his ego-ideal "I must not covet blood relations," embraces dialectically the antithetical thought of an incestuous possibility. Inasmuch as the neurotic desires to insure himself, he clings to this antithetical thought, plays with it, emphasizes it and utilizes it in the neurosis in the same way as all other frightening reminiscences which appear to him to be useful for his security. In the life of our patient, and in the lives of all neurotics, there are very many more experiences, which might have been able to carry with them

the conviction that they were free from incestuous stimuli, that they were always especially tem-
perate, careful and timorous.

Inasmuch, however, as he desires to reassure
himself, his neurotic and falsifying mode of apperception push these traits of character purposely aside. He has many more impressions to
that effect, that he does not covet his mother and
sister, but he is, however, unable to utilize them in
the service of his craving for security. Thus
there remains for them only a memory rest of a
playful preparatory venture, and because this
may serve as a warning to him, he makes of it a
bugbear, with which to frighten himself. Exactly in the same manner, develop neurotic
anxiety, fear of places, hypochondriasis, pes-
simism and constant doubting, inasmuch as these
patients only avail themselves of those impressions and experiences which serve the purpose of
bringing about security, which strengthens their
affective state while they depreciate all others
especially those of an antithetical nature. The
sophist's ability *"in utram-que partem dicere"* of
everything is also possessed by the neurotic as
well as by the psychotic, and they utilize it as
they need it.

The thoroughly polished, purposefully
strengthened dexterities of neurotics, and the
neurotic traits of character which go with them

are impossible for the fact that every new situation brings about havoc. (Lombroso's misoneismus.) More than anything else, our patient feared the, to him unknown, situation of sexual gratification and successful coitus, because in presentiments of this situation, he gave himself for reasons of safety the rôle of the underling (unterliegenden). Now this fear, which is apperceived as a fear of impotency, furnishes a further security against the possibility of being restrained, restricted in freedom or deceived by his wife, against a possibility of not being equal to her, against a rôle which is contrary to his masculine ideal, and which he therefore evaluates as effeminate.

Out of the harmless, ubiquitous traits of selfishness, avarice and stinginess, he puts together a far-reaching, apparently imminent, but in reality fictitious guiding principle of "avarice," because, the retention of this appears to him to be lost. Should he become endowed, as was the case in the dream with that which he had desired already in childhood, namely, new genitals, a healthy potency, then he must defend himself against it. He takes hold then of a means, with which he has been long acquainted, which has often been highly recommended to him, which after all enfeebles his erections instead of strengthening them,—he turns to cold washes.

This according to his experiences, inadequate remedy, he considers equal to my treatment. The remedy shall bring about the opposite to what it is aimed to do, and this physician shall have just as little success as the former ones. Thus the dream shows him the way out of the situation, it tells him how to safeguard himself against the treatment and thus get the upper hand of the physician. "Then they are second-hand goods again."

In other cases of psychic impotency a cure readily results, and as we know, as result of the most diverse kinds of remedies. Often it concerns neurotic patients who by the mere fact of going to consult a physician give one to understand that they would be inclined to give up this form of security. In that case all manner of medication, cold douches, electricity, hydrotherapy, and especially every form of suggestion, even the one resulting from an incomplete analysis are of value, occasionally the authoritative command of the physician suffices to bring about definite consequences. In severe cases, it is necessary to bring about a transformation of the all too absorbing, concentrated psyche upon the idea of security.

Age often intensely stimulates envy and avarice. Psychologically this is not difficult to understand. No matter how beautifully poets and philosophers endeavor to picture age, it is nevertheless only given to the select souls, to maintain their equilibrium, when they see looming up in the distance the gate which leads to death. Then again the denials and restrictions, which the senium naturally carries with it, and the perceptible dominancy of the younger folks, of one's own relations, which often furnish the occasion, quite innocently—or apparently so— for a degradation of old people—will almost always lead to a depression of the ego-consciousness. The sunshiny preparedness as it is refreshingly expressed in Goethe's "Father Time" is a quite unattainable illusion for most people, and fortunate indeed may be considered those who survive their best time of life without a severe depression of the spirits.

According to our thesis, it must naturally follow that the period of aging—brings forth similarly to a severe setback, a feeling of inferiority. Especially affected by this will be all those who are neurotically predisposed. At times it is age, in women, the climacteric, feelings of insufficiency of a psychic or physical nature, indications of impotency, a breaking up of the family, marriage of a son or daughter, as well as financial losses, the loss of a position or post of honor which first causes the breakdown. In most instances one may already find in the previous history indications of actual attacks of a neurotic character.

Age with its losses has the same effect as other degradations of the ego-consciousness. The aggressive tendency seeks other means whereby an adjustment may be brought about, other means which unfortunately are not easily to be had in these cases. Renunciation would come easier, if along with the sinking of bodily and mental power there would also take place a narrowing of the emotional life. This seldom happens, and in order to find a substitute for the loss, the aggressive tendency which has been stimulated by the insecurity—again whips up all stimuli of desire. The universal decree frequently stands all too firm against all these endeavors. The bearing, the life, the desires, the dress, the work and accomplishments of aging people are subject to criticism in a great measure. Those who are predisposed to a neurosis will readily take this criticism as a barricade—and will already shrink from these situations which still offer possibility of gratification. Such an individual will force himself into submission, will want to annihilate his feelings and desires, without being able to set himself to rights with them. Yes, still more intensely will these flare up when a renunciation without adjustment is demanded.

Thus it happens that the active hostile traits of character develop, that envy, ill-will, avarice, the craving for dominancy, sadistic impulses of all sorts, experience accentuations, and never satisfied, bring about a restlessness which unremittingly strives for remedies, substitutions, securities, "Where you are not—there is happiness" because the real position of aging people is seriously endangered in our state of society, inasmuch as it is the productive value, which is almost exclusively the test of the worth of the personality.   The neurotic's sustenance (Brod) on the other hand is the appearance of power, prestige, even suicide has already come within our experience as the last expression of masculine protest.

The advent of senility has even a stronger effect upon women than upon men.   Even the significance of the climacteric is usually phantastically exaggerated.   Youth and beauty meant power for woman, and more so than for man. Her charms were able to give her dominancy, victories and triumphs, for which the neurotic greediness constantly longs.

Age to them is like a stain.   Besides their value sinks more decidedly than is the case with the aging man, and as far as it concerns aging woman, prevailing psychology may be designated point blank as actually hostile.

This deplorable feature has its origin in the

well known tendency of man to depreciate woman, coupled with the psychic defeat which they experience from our social life, a neurotic germ which manifests itself, implacably and ineradicably even unto the grave. Consciously or unconsciously, often unavoidably from the nature of things, this derogatory tendency has its injurious effect upon the ego-consciousness of these aging women, who after all have a right to live. Children's love and respect for the aged as aids and guiding points of view in man's relations with his fellow men, furnish only the very minutest relief and can never suffice to gratify the stimulated desires of people whose powers are waning. It is then that the neurotic bent sets in for the purpose of strengthening the guiding principle. "I am deprimed—I had too little out of life—I will realize nothing more," this one regularly hears in the complaints of aging neurotics, and they accentuate this manner of viewing life to such an extent, that they suspiciously and distrustfully sink into a repulsive egoism, the like of which they had never before experienced so vividly. Through this, however, the vacillations and doubts become stabilized.

"Act as though you were still obliged to attain worth," thus approximately rings a newly constructed guiding principle, and along with this the nerotic's sharpening of avarice becomes more acute, the avaricious, envious, domineering impulses come violently to the foreground, almost, however, restrained by the previously mentioned guiding principles in accordance with which these patients shrink with apprehension from every desire and beginning. Thus there lie unmistakably under cover, separated with difficulty from consciousness, those impulses which lastingly support dissatisfaction, impatience, mistrust, and uninterruptedly direct the attention of the unattained and often unattainable. In the last instance, to the success of which the marked adaptability of the sexual symbols contributes in a way, but furthermore also the fact that a proof of a lack of sexual gratification is readily to be had by every one, it therefore happens, that all desire becomes sexualized. It is readily understood that these people apperceive on a sexual basis. But one must avoid taking this sexual fiction, this, so to speak, *"modus dicendi"* or as I have called it, the sexual jargon, for an original experience. In the theoretical part I have discussed the reasons for the marked prominence of the sexual guiding principle in neurotics, first, because it, like all other guiding principles is considerably accentuated in the neurotic, and so to speak, felt as real instead of what it was intended for—namely, as a protective guiding line—and second, because it (the sexual guiding principle) leads in the direction of the masculine protest.

Thus it happens that every desire of the aging neurotic woman may be referred to not only by herself, but with a little effort by the physician to a sexual analogy. Likewise, that the physician may be able to fill the neurotic's want of a protective analogy, by means of a premature offering of a sexual guiding principle in the sense of the orthodox Freudian school, may unquestionably be inferred from the foregoing considerations.

There is no gain so long as one does not succeed in ridding the patient of his fiction, which becomes possible when he becomes more certain of himself, and is able to recognize his presumably libidinous impulse as a falsifying fiction.

Such a fiction for instance is the so-called climacteric of the male, of former authors, described by Freud and Kurt Mendel. The climacteric of woman has its psychic effect irrespective of the metabolic phenomena, because of the heightening of the feeling of inferiority. Concomitant disturbances of metabolism are only able to change or intensify the neurotic's aspect, the moment it makes itself specifically felt through an intensification of the insecurity. Basedow's neurosis in climacteric women furnishes an example of such a mixed and intensified picture. The neurosis of the climacteric in man, is likewise only indirectly influenced by atrophy of the genitals, may, however, experience an intensification through the aggravating abstraction, "I am no longer a man —I am a woman." Inasmuch as the masculine guiding principle becomes intensified and hypostasized through carefulness and appropriate stimuli as a result of this ideologic standpoint those wonderful manifestations of the Johannistrieb take place, the frequent occurrence of which in women Karin Michaelis has aptly explained in her "Dangerous Age."

Only that the sexual guiding principle is not the exclusive or even most essential one as is attempted to infer from a biologic point of view, but it must be looked upon as a form of expression similar to other forms of desire if one is to face the facts squarely.

The climacteric neurosis shows us accordingly only a different phase of the neurosis caused by the masculine protest, and the traits of character demonstrable in it resemble the hypostasizations already familiar to us. I have never seen a case where the neurosis became first manifested at the climacterium. And it is to be expected according to our thesis that the "climacteric" neurosis had already shown its face in former days, at times, in a mild manner, especially when favorable circumstances or cultural activity were able to les-

sen the attack through a partial gratification of
the craving for power.   Mostly one finds a gradually progressive intensification and spreading of
the neurotic symptoms of some years duration,
which an antecedently necessitated intensification
of the craving for security permits of detection.
An example of this would be the transformation
of headache and occasional migraine into a trifacial neuralgia.   On the intensification of a neurotic cautiousness into anxiety and occasionally
through the discounting of an anticipated dis-
aster, into melancholy.   For these three steps of
protection one must consult the schema contained
in the theoretical part.

CAUTION: for instance, as if I may lose my
money, I may be beneath.

ANXIETY: as if I will lose my money, I will be
beneath.

MELANCHOLY: as if I had lost my money, as if
I were beneath.

In other words, the stronger the feeling of inferiority, the more intensified the fiction becomes
and the more closely it approaches a dogma,
through an increasing abstraction from reality.
And the patient approximates and handles everything which brings him nearer to his guiding
principle.   Reality is along with this depreciated
in various degrees, and the corrective routes become more and more inadequate.

One not infrequently sees cases in which there come to light neurotic phenomena in the pathogenic periods already known to us something on the order of an experiment. Kisch and others have called attention to this anamnestic data of neurotic complaints formed at the onset of puberty. More frequently one finds in the anamnesis neurotic molimina menstrualia, or neuroses before entering the marriage state, in the puerperium, or even continuously.

After these considerations, we shall have to let the various guiding principles described by us coördinate themselves with the prime guiding principle. The neurosis of aged people is only a different phase, an adaptive psychic superstructure built up upon the one elementary directive principle—I wish to be a man. And this directive principle, which has been outrightly condemned to destruction, avails itself of all manner of disguise, without ever finding a satisfactory one. Frequently the impression they make is one of great helplessness of resignation, as though the patient wanted to say he knew not how to go about the thing. In all their plans doubt is prominent—vacillation never leaves them, along with this, however, one sees exaggerated explanations as if the patients wished to convince themselves that they are too old, or that they are still young. The tendency is toward the gaining of power, influence, worth.   But the feeling, that they want the unattainable, never leaves them. In the dreams one regularly finds the endeavor to assist the masculine protest towards expression, to be young, to obtain sexual gratification, to show itself in a nude state, always, however, albeit at times well masked, the desire to be a man.   Also the traits of character, the secondary guiding principles, show the influence of the craving for security.

Pedantry, avarice, envy, craving for dominancy, and the desire to be popular, manifest themselves often in this disguised manner.   Anxiety is frequently found, it seems, as proof that they cannot be alone.   And in consummation, the neurotic symptoms force the entire household under the régime of the patient.   Often the attempt is made in a more or less timorous concealed manner to realize a certain wish, as though in that event the masculine protest were assured.

Frequently this wish manifests itself in a desire for divorce, or to move to a large city, or to humiliate the sons-in-law or the daughters-in-law as if tranquillity might be hoped for in that event.

Difficulties in taking food, or in emptying the bowels, or fragmentary manifestations of imaginary pregnancies and childbirths are not rare. Along with this they bring into use forgetfulness, tremulousness, here and there an occasional traumatic incident, all for the purpose of bringing to the attention of themselves and others their growing helplessness.

Complaints constantly recur, every unpleasant incident serves a special significance, and their thoughts are constantly directed toward an approaching evil. The demonstrative emphasizing of their suffering and their hesitating attitude serve on the one hand to throttle their social circle, while on the other hand it is useful for the initiation of their withdrawal from society in the event of a painful anticipation of a setback. Psychologically this complaint may also be looked upon as a form of the revolt, of the masculine protest against a feeling of inferiority, it is intended to soften and weaken those about them.

Treatment meets with considerable difficulties, inasmuch as the attainment of independence is much more difficult in advanced age, and promising predictions cannot be so plausibly made.   As always is the case, the personality of the psychotherapeutist as well as any actual or possible successes of his are utilized to spur on envy, and thus it frequently happens that improvements serve to give rise to relapses.   Then, too, the readily attainable authority over them serves to disturb the equilibrium of these patients, inasmuch as never in their life were they able to adjust them-

selves readily or what is more, subordinate themselves.   As a last refuge in severe cases, the self-
sacrifice of the physician following a thorough
analysis recommends itself, so that one is obliged
to own up to an apparent failure of his part of
the treatment, and offer the laurels to some other
therapeutic method.   In two of my cases, this
expedient justified itself, in the one case the patient, a female, was cured through the medium
of correspondence by a Bosnian country physician; in the other, a case of trifacial neuralgia
of long standing which I had been treating for
two years with varying success recovered following suggestions given against me in the wakeful
state.   In most of these cases, considerable improvement, remissions, or even complete recov-
eries set in of their own accord following the
termination of the treatment.

One of my patients, a fifty-six-year-old lady,
had been suffering for eighteen years from anxiety states, dizziness, nausea, abdominal pains
and severe obstipation.   A considerable portion
of this period was spent either in bed or lying on
a sofa, especially during the last eight years when
severe pains in the back and limbs added to her
complaints.   The patient had been previously a
robust woman but at the age of eighteen had apparently suffered for months from joint rheumatism.

Her present condition appeared to be psycho-genetic in nature, inasmuch as there was an absence of corresponding organic changes, and the protective traits of character [1] discovered by me were easily demonstrable.

The advice of a hysterectomy by a prominent gynecologist because of some perimetritic adhesions I did not take into account since I have learned to understand from other cases, the etiologic significance of such maiming procedures in the neuroses influencing as they do the psyche indirectly.

Changes, manifestations of arrests of development, deformities and disease of the genitals are frequently found in neurotics. A. Bossi certainly is correct in emphasizing this relationship as I had already done before in my "Studie" (1907). This relationship, however, lies either in the adjustment of a special feeling of inferiority which in the presence of a neurotic predisposition gives occasion for the development of a neurosis or because the neurosis, developed as result of other causes, requires a protective allusion to an organic change, in order to start upon the road the fixed goal of the masculine protest.

Sexual inferiority becomes, so to speak, the

[1] The differential-diagnostic significance of these is beyond doubt. Only one must regularly take into account the simultaneous existence of an organic affection.

vehicle which especially forces itself upon one's attention when slight changes or even wholly imagined fictitious ones such as a supposed loss of the clitoris, enlargement of the labia-majora, moistening of the apertures, telling evidences of masturbation or anomalies of the hairy growth, phimoses, paraurethral passages and asymmetric posture of the penis or testicles, or cryptorchism are taken as an occasion for a symbol of the feeling of inferiority.

This patient's disease began during a game of tennis. One year before this one of her daughters died, and her husband, a great lover of children, wished to have more children. The patient who from her earliest childhood had bewailed her lot, and wished to be a man, was not at all inclined to gratify this wish of her husband. The pain which was probably caused by a twist gave her new food for this indistinctly conscious resistance, since that time she could not stand any pressure on the abdomen, her abdomen became for her a dainty part and by means of a further bringing into use of insomnia and nausea, the latter as a memento of pregnancy, she brought matters to a point where the husband, upon the advice of physicians, abandoned sexual concourse with her, and used a separate bedroom.

Already her recital with reference to the rheumatism was characteristic. She blamed her dead mother for everything. The latter, she complained, forced her to wash and iron in the paternal home, always slighted her before the other sisters, and even in later years she was treated in the same hard-hearted manner. This woman's greediness brought her into some difficulties. But her troubles, however, she attributed to her father, so that the latter also received his share of the blame.

Such reproaches against the parents regularly draw attention according to my experience to another kind of reproach which the child is secretly making against the parents, when it finds itself incomplete, or what's more, unmanly. Such reproaches become abstract later on, as I have shown it to be likewise true of the feeling of guilt, and in later life serve the purpose, so to speak, of shells to be filled up with different content. Thus it later on sounds as if the parents were not affectionate enough, or that they pampered the child, or that especially during the masturbation period they did not supervise him sufficiently. In short, we observe in these formulations of an attitude towards the parents and later on towards the world, formal changes such as are in line with guiding principles which are to serve a practical purpose, and we frequently see a different guise cut according to the pattern of the actual situation. It is then necessary to retrace the steps covered by the formal change.   Here the analytical method makes use of the medium of reduction, of simplification (Nietzsche) of abstraction.   Along with the formal change accentuations or attenuations of the guiding fiction play an important rôle.   The more insecure the patient feels himself, the more he is driven by an unconscious tendency towards an intensification of his guiding principle, to make himself dependent upon it.   I readily follow here the worthy views of Vaihinger, who maintains for the history of ideas, that historically considered they show a tendency to grow from a fiction (an unreal but practically useful safety-device) to hypotheses and later to dogmas.   This change of intensity characterizes in a general way individual psychology, the thinking of the normal individual (fiction as an expedient) of the neurotic (attempt to realize the fiction) and of the insane (incomplete but protective anthropomorphism and realization of the fiction: dogmatization).

The stronger inner need seeks adjustment through an intensification of the assuring guiding principles.   We will therefore regularly find equivalents of the neurotics' and psychotics' guiding principles and characteristics in the normal individual, which in the latter may become corrected in order that they may be able to approach reality without contradiction.   If we were to reduce the manifest guiding principles of this patient, and free them of the various changes of form and intensity which they have undergone, so that we may take them in the original, not in the form developed later on, it would read, "I am a woman and want to be a man." The normal individual, too, adjusts himself throughout life in accordance with this formula. It aids him in attaching himself to our masculine culture, yes, it furnishes the latter with a steady impetus towards masculization (Vermännlichung). But here it plays a rôle similar to the Hilfslinie in a geometric construction. So soon as the object, a higher manly niveau is attained, it is lost from consideration (Vaihinger). Concerning the myth, a guiding principle of the race, Nietzsche laments its transformation into the fairy tale and demands a transformation into the manly (Mannliche). The neurotic emphasizes this fiction, takes it altogether too literally, and endeavors to bring about its realization.

His object is not the dovetailing, the adjustment of his masculine prestige, but to give it value, which is mostly unattainable in its overstrained form or because of intrinsic contradictions in the masculine protest, or is hindered in its attainment because of the fear of a threatening defeat, the patient still remaining ignorant of the significance and scope of his largely unconscious fiction. But his more intense feeling of uncertainty and inferiority also hinders him in the proper estimation of his fiction. The insane man conducts himself as if his fiction were a reality. He acts under the most intense urgency and delivers himself unto his self-created deity, which he apperceives as real. In a similar manner he simultaneously feels himself to be woman and superman, the latter as a reaction of the exaggerated masculine protest. The splitting of the personality corresponds to the psychic hermaphroditism, the formal change being a manifold one, manifests itself for the instant in the combination of ideas of persecution and grandeur, of depression and mania, whereas fixation as self-protection, is made facile through a relative insufficiency or absolute weakness of the corrective paths. If one were to remove from Freud's equation of dementia ("Yearbook," Bleuler-Freud, 1911) the introduced sexualization, if one were to shorten it on both sides of the superfluous libido factor, our much more profound formula of the psychic hermaphroditism with the masculine protest comes to the surface, against which, missing entirely its true significance, Freud argues in his work.

To come back to the case history, it still remains to be mentioned that our patient in her feeling of insufficiency brought forth various

forms of the masculine protest. Thus she was
unable to bring herself to remain tolerant of
men's accomplishments. In this regard, she
could be quite critical, especially when some one
tried to overestimate himself. In these cases it
not infrequently happens that physicians with a
self-confident demeanor, which appears to be an
essential to some in the treatment of disease, are
antagonized by the patient with neurotic impetu-
ousness and with the same means. In this case,
she was, aside from this, naturally guided by a
sort of instinct which forbade her to adopt the
physician's instructions, out of respect to the purpose of her disease. But at times matters reached
such a point where a harmless gain of influence
over her by the physician was responded to by
vomiting and nausea, in connection with which
the patient never missed a chance to call attention to the unsuccessful effort of the physician.
One need not lose one's tranquillity on account
of this sort of manifestation, one must rather see
in them a part of the entire whole, a formal
change of the original envy of man and later of
every one believed to be superior.

Along with this our patient made extensive use
of certain privileges given her by her illness.
First of all she was able to withdraw herself as
much as she wished to from the social duties im-

posed upon her by the rôle of housewife and important personage of a provincial city.

'Tis true she received visitors, to whom she complained of her sufferings, but only exceptionally returned a call, thus assuring herself as is the case regularly with neurotics, of a favored and privileged position.   Along with this it was possible to avoid comparisons and musterings, in one sense also trials, occasions for which social activities furnish as a rule.   Of late years she has besides been frightened by the idea that she was being robbed as a result of her growing age, of the possibilities of wielding influence over men. A lady friend demonstrated to her very intimately how ridiculously society looks upon youthful conduct in an aging woman.   Thus she decided by her way of dressing to lay special emphasis on her age, but at the same time the bitter thought crowded itself to the surface of her consciousness that men of her age are by no means pushed into the corner.

At all times she felt bitterly the fact that she had to spend her life in a provincial city.   Instinctively she strove in many ways for a removal to Vienna.   However, this was not to be attained in an open battle with her husband, who was many years her senior, because he disarmed her with his inexhaustible affection and his compliance in all other matters. She quarreled most bitterly with her brother and arranged an unbelievable anxiety of meeting this brother in this small town. When this did not suffice to bring about her object, she developed a most obstinate insomnia, as the most important cause of which she blamed the nightly rattling of wagons before the windows of her bedroom. Thus she brought about a temporary removal to Vienna, acquired a home in the neighborhood of her daughter, the heavenly peacefulness of which she constantly emphasized, and where she likewise regained her sleep.

Ever since her daughter lived in Vienna, the small provincial city became progressively more obnoxious to her. The analysis revealed in accordance with the other directive principles that she intensely envied her daughter's prestige with which there was also associated an aristocratic predicate.

She, too, wanted to live in Vienna, and would have brought this about long ago, had not a new danger threatened her in Vienna, namely, to have to cover her daughter's expenses with her own means.

The rivalry with this Viennese daughter was wholly contained in her unconscious, and corresponded with an infantile guiding line, the wish to surpass her pampered older sister. This guiding principle, too, was found to be an equivalent of the basic one, which strove toward the attainment of greater worth, as if she were a man.

On account of the heavy expenditures which her residence in Vienna imposed upon her there arose a contradiction in her masculine protest. The neurotic with his torturing feeling of inadequacy does not allow anything to be taken from him without suffering for it.

He apprehends a further belittling (Verkürzung) as a lowering of his ego-consciousness and along with his guiding principle in such a way as if this were a castration, an effeminization, a sexual assault at times also in the image of a pregnancy or birth.[2]

In our case the analogous sensations of pregnancy came especially to the surface, nausea, abdominal cramps and fixed ideas of an existing pregnancy made themselves felt, pains in the limbs represented a phlegmasia alba dolens, whereas an obstinate obstipation symbolized in part a vaginismus in the anal language, in part

[2] Thus it is that the thought process takes place not along reality, but depends on analogous symbols, whose falsifying affective accompaniment heightens the aggressive preparedness of the neurotic. The latter, however, corresponds to the unconscious, guiding "opinion." This disguise, the symbol, the analogy are as a device in the service of the aggressiveness to which the ego-ideal of the neurotic compels.

The woman as a Sphinx, the man as a murderer, etc.

attempting to prevent expenditures symbolically, and thirdly attempted to express the impossibility of an independent conduct.

A more profound understanding of the mode of expression of the neurosis appears to me to be impossible without the knowledge of the "organ-jargon" discovered by me. Folklore takes cognizance of this in the expression of popular speech and custom. Freud misunderstood this jargon, and has created out of its constructions the mainstay of his libido-theory, namely the theory of the erogenous zones. Especially his work on the anal character and analerotic is full of a strained and overworked phantasy. The point of outset is the relative inferiority of certain organs, the attitude of the environment towards the manifestations of these organs as well as the mass-impressions of the two upon the soul of the child. Neurotically predisposed children will endeavor to associate with suitable manifestations of their organ-inferiority especially with defects of childhood, those traits of character which have their origin in their protesting ego-consciousness, such as obstinacy, greater need of affection, exaggerated cleanliness, pedantry, anxiousness, ambition, envy, revengefulness, etc., in order to gain an especially effective representation. One of my psychogenic epileptics utilized for the purpose of strengthening his masculine protest such a device, an interlacing, so to speak, inasmuch as he managed to have most of his attacks preceded by an attack of obstipation in order to arouse anxious forebodings in his relatives and thus bring himself to their notice in the event of a degradation.

Obstinacy and infantile negativism may already be well developed towards the end of the nursing period. It is the association of these anomalies of urination, defecation, and eating, which gives rise to the heightened "reasoning." The child who abstains from emptying his bowels derives his pleasurable sensations not from an irritation of the rectum, but from the satisfaction of his obstinacy which avails itself of this unesthetic means, but may, however, attribute a pleasure-quality to rectal sensations for years, up to the curing of his obstinacy.

The mother of a nearly two-year-old girl who was still suffering from bed-wetting told me that she had frequently observed that when awakened from her sleep her child would attend properly to the emptying of the bladder, providing she was still in a half-wakeful state only, but no sooner did she become fully awake than she refused to do so. If the child became fully awake towards the end of urination, she upset the urinal and cried a long time out of rage at being thus taken unawares; if, on the other hand, she still continued half asleep she turned over and went fast asleep.

Thus we may find in every case that from the very earliest period of existence the ego-consciousness of the child finds itself in a manifest and latent contrast with its environment, that it assumes a most pronounced attitude of hostility and belligerency until it finally brings about a uniform termination of all these aggressive stimuli, until it constructs these into the masculine protest which it brings in opposition to the stimuli of tenderness, subordinacy, and weakness, as well as to the manifestations of inferiority, all of which it collectively apperceives and combats as symptoms of femininity. Only that at times an interlacing and intertwining takes place, where the masculine protest lays stress upon feminine symptoms in order to utilize them as a bugbear, or where he obstinately retains feminine symptoms and this makes possible the development of hermaphrodistic constructions which likewise exert their influence in the direction of the masculine protest. For example, tears, indispositions, simulations and exaggerations of childhood defects. The overaccentuated guiding principle, namely, "I wish to be a man," enlists then within its ranks all utilizable bodily symptoms, particularly those manifestations of inferiority upon which the attention of the patient as well as that of the environment is especially directed.

Thus it happens that the masculine protest makes use of a "somatic language" for the purpose of gaining expression. A beautiful example, one which frequently recurs in neurotic phantasies is that of Leonardo da Vinci's childhood phantasy: "A vulture repeatedly shoved its tail into his mouth." This phantasy carries the artist's psychic constellation to a most accurate abstraction. Mouth phantasies are regularly related to manifestations of inferiority in the child's gastro-intestinal tract. Leonardo's inclinations to a science of nutrition were most likely the fruits of the attention directed to these channels.

The tail of the vulture is a phallic symbol. A summing up of these two trends brings forth the characteristic basic idea, "I will experience the lot of the woman." But this rigid adherence to a symbolic guiding principle already draws our attention to the fact that these and similar trends of thought do not signify a psychic settlement but serve, under the pressure of our masculine culture, for a heightened impetus in the opposite direction, must lead to an over compensation toward the masculine side, where they evolve the masculine guiding principle the more distinctly, "therefore I must act in such a manner as if I were a complete man."

That these two guiding principles contradict

one another, aside from the fact that each individually is a contradiction to reality, in so far as they are taken literally and not as something useful and corrigible, I have already set forth in my contribution on the "Psychic hermaphroditism in life and in the neurosis" ("Fortschritte der Medizin," Leipzig, 1908).

This contradiction is reflected in doubt, in indecision, and in fear of making decisions, the analysis of which reveals more or less the fact that there existed in early childhood an uncertainty as to the future sexual rôle, in the psychic superstructure of which all later sensations, feelings and stimuli were grouped in a certain sense as doubtful, "I don't know whether I am a man or a woman" (see "Predispositions to Neurosis," Year Book, Bleuler-Freud, 1909).

Our patient expressed in the anal language that she had closed up an opening. A distinctly feminine thought. One may picture to himself a group of men and women dressed in women's clothes gathered in a room into which a mouse was suddenly let loose. The women will at once betray their sex in that they will draw their clothes around their legs, as if they tried to prevent the mouse from entering. In the same manner, the feminine frightening guiding principle is betrayed by a fear of holes, of being bitten, stabbed, ideas of persecution by men, by bulls, the position of the back, the being pulled to the right, backwards, to be pressed upon, to fall, etc., a guiding principle which is readily reacted to with an insuring anxiety.[3]

Obstipation as a neurotic symptom takes its origin in a hereditary defect of the intestines, which leads to a neurotic closure of the sphincter through ideas concerning anal birth and sexual relation. As a matter of fact this patient suffered in her childhood from intestinal catarrh and occasional intestinal incontinence, later from obstipation and a recto-vaginal fistula.

That the closure of the anus was under the domination of a guiding idea of closing of cavities is likewise seen from the fact that the patient suffered for a considerable length of time following her marriage from vaginismus. The obstipation of this aging woman expresses in a dual way the same desire as did her erstwhile vaginismus, namely, "I don't want to be a woman, I want to be a man."

At this point I must for practical, as well as for theoretical reasons go considerably beyond the scope of a mere character delineation, as one is for that matter usually compelled to take into account the psyche as a whole in every discussion

---

[3] The same masculine protest leads in the neurosis to trismus, blepharospasmus, vaginismus, spasm of the sphincter, globus and spasm of vocal cords.

of psychological questions. Besides this so minutely analyzed case furnishes a clearer insight than it is possible to gain in other cases, especially where because of a dependence upon the physician or upon extraneous circumstances a cure or discontinuance of the treatment takes place before the scheme, according to which the patient built his psychosis, becomes completely revealed. Thus I will attempt to set forth in this case, this scheme, by arranging according to this analytically disclosed scheme all her symptoms, the sentinels opposite the outer world, and show the synthetic relationship of the traits of character with it.

According to this scheme (p. 184–6) the patient arranged all her experiences, and wherever they fitted at all, occasion for which is amply furnished in the life of every individual by his symbolic as well as purposive apperceptions, she reacted to them with the appropriate disease manifestations. The protective traits of character were pushed to the fore, like outposts, were ever ready for defense, and explained situations in accordance with guiding thoughts, and whenever the occasion arose, borrowed support from the sum total of the appropriate symptoms. Her manifestations of independence were considerably interfered with by the intelligent and tender attitude of her husband and by certain benevolent guiding principles of the patient. Thus it happened that the basic scheme, "I'm only a woman," derived its influence from intentionally retained impressions of the feminine rôle, in connection with which the unconscious mechanism of the masculine guiding thoughts furnished the protecting memento. The healthy woman is characterized by a more conscious attitude toward the feminine rôle by a purposive dovetailing and corrective approximation of the scheme to reality. The psychosis produced an accentuation of the imaginary scheme for protective purposes, and an incorrigible attitude within this scheme; such a patient will conduct herself as if she really were pregnant. In all three cases the fiction of pregnancy and the greater circle of its manifestations, a symbol of the inferior feminine rôle, a convincing expression for the feeling of degradation, but at the same time looked upon from the standpoint of the masculine protest, an artifice for the purpose of avoiding further degradation, as was shown above.[4]

[4] The transformation of the masculine fiction may reach a point where under its direction maternity, pregnancy, may be striven for, quite frequently in such cases where obstacles of a very gross nature exist. The cry for a baby is then regularly directed against the man. Phantom pregnancies frequently represent such an arrangement.

SCHEME

SYMPTOMS

Fear of society.	The leaning from the feminine rôle, the masculine protest.	Protective dexterities. ——— Mistrust (credulity with subsequent protest).
Compulsive blushing		
Fear of being alone. Palpitation of the heart. Fear of falling, dizziness when in high places.	Protection against courting.	Belittling of man. Anxiousness. Bashfulness (timidity). Virtuous morality. Desire to dominate (submission with subsequent protest).
Feeling of pressure in the stomach. (Cæcum.) Frigidity. Overacuity of hearing of husband's snoring. Vaginismus, pressure sensations over the breasts.	Protection against coitus.	Willfulness. Obstinacy.

Inability to stand any kind of pressure, the struggle against the corset. A feeling of being drawn to the right and downward (towards the feminine side). Noises in the ears. (The noise of the moving sea, which swells and falls.)	Protection against coitus.	Disputatiousness. Tendencies hostile to the husband.
Abdominal pains. Shortness of breath. Palpitation of the heart. Nausea. Vomiting. Compulsory ideas of pregnancy. Fatigue. Craving for certain foods.	Protection against pregnancy.	Somatic oversensitiveness. Hypochondriacally to pamper oneself.
Abdominal cramps. Difficult evacuation of the bowels, signifying difficult labor. Occasional polyuria. (Passing of the waters.)	Protection against parturition.	

Objection to lying on bed.
Pain in legs.
Tendency to prolong invalidism.
} A fiction of a thrombophlebitis
} Protection against puerperium.

Form of action of a complex type for the purpose of doing away with the inferiority and degradation.

Weakness in limbs, reminding one of astasia and abasia.
Staggering gait.
Easy fatiguibility in walking.
} A memento of leaving the childbed.

Avarice, thriftiness, envy, desire to dominate, impatience, fear of attaining nothing, of completing nothing, all sorts of exertions, as if the distance toward equality with men were to be diminished in any possible way.

A hostile, at times sadistic behavior towards children.
Rapid fatiguing, tiring and impatience in the care of children.
Insomnia.
Finickiness in matters of cleanliness.
Over-acuteness of hearing at night.
Light sleeping.
} Protection against maternal duties.

A dream which took place towards the end of the treatment shows us the original guiding thought of the patient in connection with her actual inner conflicts. She dreamed: *"As if she were sitting on a bench in a park near the residence of her parents, ill and weak. She wore on her head two bathing caps. Two girls then approached from behind her and one of them tore one of the caps from her head. She grabbed hold of the girl and held her while the other one disappeared and threatened to report her to the police. A poor, badly clothed woman passed by and told her that the girl's name was Velicka. At this point she went to her mother in order to complain. Her mother gave her a basket full of eggs and said they cost 5 guldens. She took two of the eggs in her hand and saw that they were pretty."*

The situation on the bench; her fatigue and the bathing caps referred to a hydropathic treatment which she had undertaken especially for the removal of an insomnia prior to coming under my care. On the day preceding the dream she reprimanded her daughter because the latter used her bath linen for her own use; she also possessed two bathing caps, as in the dream, which the daughter likewise often used. Velicka is a Slavic word signifying big. The daughter had a Slavic "Adelspraedikat." The poorly-dressed woman is a noblewoman by the name of Grand-venire. Opposed to the two is she, the plebeian, degraded one. She was dissatisfied because her husband was not knighted, but on account of her pride she did not acknowledge this envy. She was afraid that the daughter might be able to take everything away from her. She had two daughters, one died, disappeared. She often complained to me that her daughter cost her much money. She has already given her all her jewelry. From her very childhood she has always been degraded before others. Even her mother always humbled her and demanded payment from her for every little thing after the patient had become married. She, on the other hand, supplied her daughter regularly with eggs, venison, milk, butter, etc., and still she needed so much money. Before she left for Vienna she forgot to settle a debt of 5 guldens. The day previous she wrote to her husband that he should pay this at once. In fact she always had to pay at once for everything she bought.[5]

The mother treated her badly. In the dream she recalled a forgotten obligation. She always

[5] The fear to become humiliated through further expenses is closely allied to the utilization of the character-type of greed and parsimony. These maternal, and according to her way of looking, feminine traits, she avoided through a compulsion to pay beforehand and showed herself to be superior to her mother through her liberality.

saved at her expense. In the dream she received from her mother the masculine attribute (testicles) which the mother kept from her at the time of birth. We see again how out of the feeling of femininity (degradation) the masculine protest is in the dream directed against further insults. This dream shows us the attempt of the patient to evade in her thoughts further degradation and to accuse her daughter that like her mother she kept everything from her.

Similarly, this lust to possess everything is found in the following case history which shows still more clearly than the preceding case how the patient on account of his pride seeks to remove this lust from his field of vision, to repress it. We shall see how a decided change takes place through the revelation of this repression and through the elucidation of the Œdipus complex. In the same manner it appears from all these cases that this lust to have everything pursues the most senseless goals. Such patients have eyes for everything which others in their circle possess in so far as they are excluded from the possession of the same. They may possess more than the others and yet they will envy them. They may gain everything which they formerly begrudged others and will then unceremoniously set it aside in order to furnish new goals for their desires and possessions. And their lust for possession ever remains attached to those goals which they have not attained. It is readily understood that they are incapacitated for love and friendship. Often they acquire a general ability to misrepresent and set out to captivate souls because others also dominate. They constantly fear degradation and always seek to assure themselves long beforehand. The love of the parents enjoyed by the brother, their jewelry, the marriage of a brother or of a sister, a book, an accomplishment of an acquaintance or even of a total stranger, fill them with rage.[6]

The superiority of another, a successfully passed examination, possession or worth of brothers and sisters throw them into excitements, cause them headache, insomnia and more pronounced neurotic symptoms. Their constant fear not to become the equal of an older or younger brother may render them unfit for work. It is then that they attempt to avoid all decisions and tests, it is then that they reach the stage of loss of initiative, approach often in any possible way the withdrawal from life and support themselves in the meanwhile on their *ad hoc* created symptoms among which there came to my atten-

[6] Thus an approaching marriage of a girl may lead to the development of a neurosis in the brother or father when the latter are neurotically disposed. Thus the arrangement of affection may then give the impression of incest stirrings.

tion frequently compulsory blushing, migraine, all sorts of headaches, palpitation of the heart, stuttering, agoraphobia and claustrophobia, tremor, sleepiness, depression, weakness of memory, excessive thirst and psychogenic epilepsy.

I have especially emphasized above the case of the younger brother because I met with him oftenest and because he is most apt to be driven to rivalry.[7] This case is not an exception. One also finds in this rôle older siblings or only children, naturally also girls. The rivalry may also be directed primarily against the father or mother in whose picture the desired superiority appears to be concretely represented. It is then that the Œdipus-complex develops out of the longing of the predisposed child, as a guiding model, a guiding fiction to gain satisfaction for his craving, and this takes place at a time when sexual craving is still out of the question, but it is also the desire to possess a person or an object which belongs to another. A belief in predestination and ideas of identification with God frequently develop as manifestations of the masculine protest. Kleptomania is frequently revealed in the anamneses of these patients. At times the patient is unconscious of his guiding principle. Occasionally he is seen at work trying to conceal this guiding prin-

[7] Frischauf, "Psychology of the Younger Brother." Munich, A. Reinhardt, 1912.

ciple and to make it unrecognizable through a manifestation of opposed tendencies such as liberality.

The wish which, for instance, draws him to his mother, changes nothing after it has become conscious in the disease-picture, no matter how frankly sexual it may be shown to be. It is only after the patient understands and controls his desire for the unattainable, for that which in the nature of things belongs to another, that recovery may take place.

The boundless pride which one detects in some of these cases does not readily permit the patient to gain insight into his envy and jealousy. The tendency to belittle others is, on the other hand, quite markedly developed and readily comes to the surface. Malice, revengefulness, desire for intrigue (and in those of lower intelligence), more crudely aggressive tendencies, even sadistic and murder-instincts reveal themselves as attempts to insure oneself against a degradation in this eternal rivalry. The fear of the consequences, such as a lively concern about the needs of relatives, the picturing to oneself of punishments, arrest and misery are appertaining assurances against the ebullitions of the masculine protest. Even epileptic seizures may serve as security devices, thus, for instance, as in our case, where a psycho-epileptic insult associated itself with patricidal and fratricidal dream-stir-rings.

It is possible that the motive of a "scorned love" regularly plays a rôle in these cases, and brings about the most intense hate against the un-attained person. One may justly doubt whether love in a normal person is capable of such a trans-formation. It requires the sum-total of power-instincts, the over-heated ego-consciousness of these individuals to desire to bring about the spir-itual possession of another person against that person's will. Inasmuch as the neurotic desires to possess everything, he is blind to all natural restrictions, and experiences in the scorn of his love a thrust at his most sensitive principle. Now he turns to revenge: *Acheronta movebo.*

When one is in doubt as to which of two per-sons the patient has selected for his affections, whether the father or mother, it is safe to assume that it is the opposite to the one the patient men-tions. It would be too painful, as a rule, to ac-knowledge scorned love. An exact solution seems to me to be furnished by the following sim-ple experiment:

One places the patient exactly between the two persons in question, and soon one observes that he has moved nearer the preferred one.

Thus I was able to discover in the case which I am about to discuss in detail that the patient

showed decided preference for his mother, though
when he was alone he always gave preference to
his father. He not infrequently scolded his
mother, and not a day passed but what they quarreled.

A certain manifestation which one frequently
observes in the neuroses was likewise present
here, and in an especially accentuated form,
namely, the strong emphasis of a pedantic character trait, which, not unlike the "crack regi-
ment" in war time, took over the task of coming
in touch with the enemy. The enemy was first
of all the mother, and the daily battles regularly
developed because the latter was unable to do full
justice to the patient's pedantic demands in eating, in dressing, in the preparation of his bath or
bed. Our patient thus gained a base of operation—from which emanated the various subterfuges by means of which he endeavored to place
his mother, after all, completely at his service.
In this is seen again a neurotic trait of character
as a device, by means of which the patient seeks
to be true to his inner fiction, to dominate his
mother in the same manner as he believed to have
observed his father dominate her. "And should
you be unwilling, I'll use force." This train of
thought gained stability from the patient in his
youth, and thus he at once assumed towards his
mother an attitude full of mistrust, constantly

on the alert for setbacks, for the preferring of others, full of tense energy and gloomy expectation whether he will yet succeed in gaining her for himself. Not because he really loved her, or really desired to possess her, but because his desire for possession of her was similar to the desire which he had for many other things, jewelry, bonbons, which he valued not at all highly, but left lying in a drawer, forgotten, once he could call them his own. Thus the possession of the mother was not an end in itself, his desire was not at all a libidinous or sexual one, but the mother and his distance from her became a symbol for him, an estimate of his own inferiority. And because he apperceived the cosmic picture, every new acquaintance, every relation to the opposite sex with the same traits of character, suspiciously, full of sensitiveness, with a similar expectation of a disappointment, all success fled from him, all satisfaction in life was lost to him. He had eyes only for everything which spoke against him, against his success, and whatever he did attain lost all charm for him. He settled the problem of his life with the arrangement of his neurosis. He considered himself deficient by a whole lot— and this deficiency was represented in the symbolic loss of the mother.

Does one suppose that this patient who had been suffering from anxiety-states, migraine and depressions, could have been cured if his mother were returned to him? Such an attempt would have been fruitless at the time the patient came to the physician. Even the most compliant mother—and many of them are lastingly estranged from their sons—could not have shown that measure of patience and sacrifice which the patient demanded in his boundless mistrust and desire for dominancy. The past, and the thought of former privations, were ever ready to furnish motives for new outbreaks and oppres-- sions. It is possible that the attempt at cure might have been a successful one in the patient's childhood, a pedagogic solution of this special neurotic problem in a gradual orientation and independence of the child, and an appropriate tranquilizing of the child concerning his future. It is the *uncertainty* which mars the outlook for the future in these children, an uncertainty whose organic and psychic roots we already know. In our case it was the fact that the patient, already as a child, even during the suckling period showed a tendency to become easily frightened and panicky. This fright of sucklings—which is frequently taken as nervousness—is obviously an organic inheritance and is associated, according to my observations, with an hereditary sensitive- ness, inferiority of the auditory apparatus, so that children already become panicky in the presence of noises and tones to which other children pay no unusual attention. From our standpoint this striking tendency to fright signifies a sign of an hereditary, auditory oversensitiveness, a manifestation of a somatic inferiority of the familiar ear diseases, but likewise corresponds to a heightened refinement of hearing in the musical sense. The fact that our patient suffered at the age of 6 years from a protracted middle ear disease which necessitated paracentesis of the ear drum, is in accord with our views concerning somatic inferiority; similarly, his development of an excellent musical ear and of a strikingly refined sensitiveness in hearing which especially qualified him for eavesdropping. This somatic refinement brings with it that the child is driven to a development of a tendency towards a lurking curiosity, even though he may feel more marked uncertainties from other causes. The roots of this uncertainty from which he endeavors to escape by means of his curiosity, laid in the patient's weaker intellect, compared with an older brother —who as it often happens to the detriment of bringing up—made of the patient the plaything of his railleries and often made a fool of him.

The patient also recalled to have suffered from that form of cryptorchism in which a testicle occasionally disappears into the abdominal cavity through the patent canal. This fact, that is, the better sexual development of his brother, the earlier maturity of the latter, brought to his mind quite early the thought that he is perhaps a girl after all.   Up to the fourth year of his life he was dressed in girls' clothes, and during this period he developed the fear that he never perhaps would reach the mature state of his father or his older brother, that is, never become a complete man. The marked development of his breasts lent considerable weight to his uncertainty.   That he unconsciously gave considerable thought to the question of the difference of the sexes, one may glean from an occurrence which remained fixed in his memory, because at the time he told it every one laughed at him.   One day while in a public park he watched a girl urinate and upon reaching home related how he had seen a boy urinate from behind.[8]

This early period in his life was of marked significance in shaping his attitude towards his family and in a broader sense to the world at large. He saw himself belittled, and his feeling of inferiority found no adjustment in the family.   His covetousness, his craving to become the equal of

[8] The original uncertainty of the sexual rôle, as I have been emphasizing for years, plays one of the chief parts in the development of the neurotic psyche, which is later on vitalized as a symbol and base of operation in the struggle for dominancy. It is only of late that many authorities are beginning to agree with me on this point.

his brother, of his father, of anyone whom he considered strong, able, powerful, gained in intensity and directed him upon paths in which he came into serious conflicts with his parents. He became a bad, unmanageable child, which made a tender attitude of his parents towards him still more difficult. His desires assumed measureless proportions, he began to insure himself against every setback suspiciously and with a growing choler, and this at a time when his maturing genitalia, his strikingly hairy body, his improved insight into matters sexual, should have had their tranquilizing effect upon him. But by this time his position in the family became such an unfavorable one, owing to the development of his traits of character, which likewise unfavorably influenced his school work, that with his over-sensitive nature he had good reason to feel himself slighted and belittled. Thus he was no longer able to find the road to normality. That he, however, continued to apperceive this slight—in the manner of an analogy with the feminine rôle—became already evident from the first dream which he recited during the treatment. The dream was *"I felt as if I were witnessing an ape nursing a child."*

His brother often called him an ape because of his excessive hairy growth, which he nevertheless exhibited with pride. The ape, which is

nursing the child, a female ape, is he himself—
that is, he sees himself, he feels himself in a feminine rôle, along with which the nursing is to be
considered a gynecomastia ("Gynakomastie")
which came up during the dream analysis. This
is the feminine principle emphasized by me for
all dreams—against which the stressing of the
excessive hairy growth is to be understood as
pointing in the direction of the masculine protest. Thus the patient enters upon the treatment with the disclosure that he feels himself belittled—and permits us to divine from the choice
of his figure of speech, that he evaluates this inferiority as feminine.

I wish to draw attention, in this connection, to
the fact that the dreamer often chooses pictures
and forms of expression which show a simultaneous coloring of feminine and masculine traits.
Here it was an ape, whose nursing was a feminine
characteristic, while the hairy growth is to be
apperceived as a masculine characteristic. Such
forms of expression which I have recognized as
belonging to the psychic hermaphroditism may be
referred to two simplifying circumstances.
First, they correspond to the infantile indefinite-
ness of sex-cognition. Second, because the element of time, as in other cases, the element of
space, is during the marked abstraction of the
dream state wholly or almost wholly eliminated,

so that his thoughts which may be separated spatially or temporally, become united—in one case the thoughts were "I feel myself a woman and wish to be a man." Stekel, in his further elaboration of my conception of psychic hermaphroditism, assumes a double sexual meaning for every dream symbol, which I think is a certain exaggeration, nevertheless he comes closer to the truth than does Freud who denies the regular manifestation in the dream of psychic hermaphroditism and the masculine protest.

The distinctness with which this first dream of our patient points to his feeling of inferiority, so to speak, in the form of a reaction to the beginning of the treatment, is naturally also to be understood as an omen for the benefit of the physician:—"My disease has its origin in my feeling of inferiority."—"My disease," fainting attacks and business incapacity are security devices against a defeat in the fifth act. "I am impotent and inefficient as a child and long for love, apelove, as I see it in the dream." We fill out:— impotent for reason, in order to be pampered like a child, which he succeeds in attaining more readily after his attacks; and inefficient, in order that he may always be supplied with maintenance, in order that it may not be forgotten that he must be made secure for life through affection and legacy. His marked tendency to be frightened by sudden noises, his hyperacusis was especially fitted to aid him in gaining his point. The finale which he set before him, a desired over-compensation for a feeling of inferiority, consisted in not more nor less than the desire to gain the love of his parents, especially that difficult of attainment, mother's love. Thus he utilizes, with the object of influencing his mother's heart, the already-mentioned experiences, such as becoming frightened upon hearing a shot, as he often manifested upon hearing the firing at a military funeral, upon hearing the puffing and shrill whistling of a locomotive, and during a sudden assault by his brother or playmates. The finale which constantly stands before his eyes, drew upon itself a fixation of this hyperacusis, which dominated him up to the present. This purposeful hypersensitiveness serves, as do similar phenomena in hysteria, to show us that the patient's uncertainty forces him to stretch forth his antennæ as far as possible, as he is actually doing with over-tense traits of character. Aside from this his tendency to fear pressed upon his masculine feeling and gave him the sense of feminine stimuli. He endeavored, therefore, to bring forth in all other relations, courage and fearless behavior, in which he succeeded too.

The laying bare of his desire for the love of the mother brought forth no particular result. His attacks occurred at about the same intervals, but now he had them in bed, in order to protect himself in this way from the possible inroads of the treatment, which, at this stage, was encountering more difficulty in endeavoring to uncover the causes of his attacks. Prior to this the attacks occurred always in connection with experiences which threatened him with a set-back, but now I was compelled to reconstruct these experiences from his thoughts and dreams. Naturally the patient made a virtue of this necessity, and spoke of this change as an improvement due to my treatment, thus expecting to gain in this way my sympathy, an experience which he always apperceived as a feeling of power. To this craving after this feeling of power he owes his success in passing as a very sociable and pleasant fellow in his intercourse with strangers.

It may be spoken here that because of my different conception of these matters, the Œdipus-complex does not come very clearly to the surface, here, at any rate not so clearly as Freud has demonstrated this complex. To this I would have to object energetically. It was this case particularly, as so few of them are, which brought to view regardless of consequence, the striving for the mother in a sexual manner, and the patient at no time hesitated to elaborate the frequently unconcealed Œdipus dreams as proof of his sexual striving after his mother. He had many such dreams. He dreamed: *"I'm walking with a lady from our rendezvous towards the street."*

The lady represented his mother, as the various details showed. The "street" referred to prostitution. The "rendezvous" on the other hand was a memory-remnant from his waking life and referred to a girl who refused him another meeting, thus by her refusal simulating his mother. He was unable to wield any influence over girls, and was thus, according to his own understanding, driven to the masculine—feeling of power—and in his protest degraded to the level of a prostitute his mother as well as the girl, and for that matter all women whom he naturally feared.

Just as clearly the Œdipus-complex came to light in other dreams, where too the sexual, as a jargon, as a mode of speech, was only recognized after a penetration into the psychic constellation. Thus he dreamed: *"I'm sitting at a smooth table made of brown wood. A girl brings me a large vessel of beer."* The table reminded him of a subterranean cellar at Nüremberg, where he went to attend a scientific undertaking which led him to the German museum. His thoughts drifted in the same general direction of Germanism in connection with the large vessel of beer. It is quite comprehensible that this unusually musical patient should in the analysis come upon Wagner's "Meistersinger." As he mentioned this he began to search for a scene in Wagner's operas, wherein some one takes a drink. At first he thought of Tristan, then of Siegfried's arrival at Gunter's palace. In both scenes the hero drinks a love potion. Thus our patient apperceives his enigmatical attraction for his mother as something provoked by the mother's magical powers. At last he thought of Siegmund whom his sister Sieglinde compassionately gives a horn of meal.

Thus the dream reads:—The voice of blood (relation) hath spoken, the mother compassionately takes his part, he is the hero, who is the man (father) of his wife. An incestuous prospect, as in Wagner, the patient, as if intoxicated, longs after his mother.

The psychic situation of the patient had experienced an "effeminization." His older brother had returned from a journey and was welcomed at home with much love. How different were matters upon his own return from his travels in Germany. The thought, I am belittled, became accentuated through the reception accorded his brother, and in the dream he seeks to save himself through a masculine guiding line. It was an attempt which was bound to fail. The same night he had a seizure.

The seizure had for its purpose the direction of the mother's tenderness towards the patient.

This was quite successful with the father. But even the mother would forget his jealous, frequently vulgar outbreaks of temper, as soon as he lay unconscious, and for a time would sit on his bed. Thus he satisfies his wish, his wish to possess everything, like the brother, like the father. The change of form of his original fiction, namely —I have imperfect genitalia, I will not be a complete man— had reached the thought, I too wish to possess my mother as my father and brother possess her. In order to comport himself in this matter with the appropriate amount of energy, it required a deeply-felt conviction of his longing for his mother, which he proceeded to create.

The most essential reason for his ardent attitude towards his mother was revealed in the further analysis, which revealed as the decisive point his feeling of uncertainty. As the mother isolated herself more and more from him during his childhood, he developed the idea, as is the case not infrequently with such children, that he did not belong to his family. The fairy tales of "Snow White" and "Cinderella" frequently furnish these children with leading thoughts. When his brother was ill once the mother did not leave him for a second. Since then the patient was uninterruptedly stimulated to test, by means of his severe seizures, the family, especially the mother, and see if the "voice of blood" will speak.

These tests he carried out with a genuine neurotic insatiability, and thus we see also in this case that the Œdipus-complex is of the nature of an especially arranged fiction, utilized as a means of expression for the masculine protest against a feeling of uncertainty and inferiority, and dependent upon the neurotic craving for security, the desire to possess everything.

The inner contradiction which frequently comes into being in this form of masculine protest, the moral condemnation of a conduct corresponding to the basic thought "to possess everything," but also the greater insight into the impossibility of attainment or the fear of a decision which may assail the patient often necessitate a compromise. This may best be expressed by the words "half and half." The patient seeks a way out of this dilemma and thus reaches the point of *"divide et impera."* At times this solution is tenable, because of the possibility of a gratification of the desire for dominancy.

At times this leads to a marked cultural but also utopian development of feeling of equality and love for justice.

CHAPTER II

THE NEUROTIC EXTENSION OF LIMITS THROUGH
ASCETICISM, LOVE, DESIRE TO TRAVEL, CRIME.
SIMULATION AND NEUROSIS. FEELING OF IN-
FERIORITY OF THE FEMALE SEX. PURPOSE OF
AN IDEAL. DOUBT AS AN EXPRESSION OF PSY-
CHIC HERMAPHRODITISM. MASTURBATION
AND NEUROSIS. THE INCEST-COMPLEX AS A
SYMBOL OF CRAVING FOR DOMINANCY. THE
NATURE OF THE DELIRIUM. (Delirium used
in the sense of the French: UNE DELIRE.)

A CONSIDERATION which should align itself here
endeavors to show how the compensating guiding
idea, "to possess everything" may deviate from its
straight course in order to stimulate in a round-
about way or by means of an artifice accomplishments of a strangely neurotic, criminal, but also
of a creative kind, in order to reach its ultimate
good eventually and bring about in some way a
maximation of the ego-consciousness or at least—
and to this extent the neurosis remains productive—to prevent a degradation.

The parsimony, penury and asceticism of certain neurotics already shows us such a detour

upon which the patient permits himself to be driven as if he were able to avoid danger only in this way. He then behaves strictly according to these guiding ideas, believes in them and accentuates his abnormal being in moments of especial uncertainty to the point of a psychosis. In melancholic states when poverty phantasies predominate, as well as in hypochondriacs, the patient in order to avoid the real danger, anticipates the feared state, endeavors to realize a fiction, emphasizes his feeling of inferiority and utilizes his disease for the safeguarding of his ego-consciousness. Cases exhibiting the lying-mania, fetichism, neurotic mania for gathering up things and kleptomania, also illustrate this craving to possess everything. Another evident trait exists, namely, to break through the boundaries laid down by reality in the direction of a fictitious guiding principle, in order to escape a feeling of degradation. Apperception always comes to light according to the rigidly formal antithesis of "manly-womanly" and frequently leads the patient to undertake accentuations by means of which it may be proved that he is a man. Sexual symbolism lends itself very well as a means of expression for this purpose, the solution of which is at times furnished by the exaggerated masculine trend through peculiar detours. Here belongs the neurotic lying, braggardism, as well as attempts to play with fire and love and thus extend as far as possible the established limits. Less harmful manifestations are pathological wanderlust, the expression of which is to be seen in the running away, in the fugues of neurotic and psychotic subjects. As a rule there exists in the guiding picture of these neurotics an ideal of personality, the apex of which it is attempted to reach through imitation or obstinate, negativistic behavior. The same trend, namely, to extend masculine cognition, to its very limits, is at the bottom also of the constant tendency to read about, listen to, see and commit acts of a disgusting nature.

The more pronounced this striving for worthless possession, the more normal tendencies and values are falsified, similarly to the manner in which love for nature is only a deception, but furnished in an exaggerated manner, when a tourist wants to have every peak noted upon his mountain staff.

The Leporelist shows us this desire with reference to love and the Messalina is to be compared with Don Juan, a nymphomaniac who always imagines herself unsatiated and belittled because in this neurotic form real possibilities for gratification are unattainable. The fettering and degradation of the partner are of course taken into consideration in this relation.

"Dear soul, what place can you think of where I have not been?" Immermann's Munchausen answers to the question, whether he knew a certain distant place. The real satisfaction in active games, riding, driving, racing and aviation originate, from the desire for possession, for conquest. For this reason every child aspires to be a coachman, a conductor, a locomotive engineer or an aviator, but to no less an extent he wishes to be emperor or teacher in order to command his companions and to find a visible expression for his superiority, or a physician in order to conquer death and to extend the limits of life, or a general in order to lead an army or an admiral in order to command the sea. Lies, thefts and other crimes committed by children are manifestly attempts to extend the limits of power in this way. For the most part these attempts assume no more real form than that of day dreams or phantasies. An inquiry instituted by me in a girls' high school showed that all of the twenty-five girls remembered having committed trivial thefts. I was able to include even the teacher. On closer examination the motive for this striving for attainment is the intolerable stimulus arising from the child's feeling of inferiority. Frequently the child under this pressure is curious, eager to learn, seeks to recognize his faults and to make for himself a place for unfolding his personality.

Defects, misfortunes, the feeling of uncertainty and inferiority often force a strong development of the higher psychic faculties, analogous to the compensatory stress in the organic compensatory tendency. Jatgeir says in Ibsen's "Pretender to the Crown," "I received the gift of pain and became a skald." It is easy to prove in a number of cases that a particularly strong feeling of inferiority sets into activity the impulse to investigation, or that the "vocation" to the life of an artist which later presents the example of a harmonious accord of art and life "began with a crude dissonance" (B. Litzmann, Clara Schumann).

Another way in which children often show themselves superior to their parents has been described by me in the "Psychic Treatment of Trigeminal Neuralgia." This may consist in the following: From memory of earlier defects in imitation of others, a state of apparent stupidity, blindness, deafness, limping, stuttering, enuresis, untidiness, awkwardness, lack of appetite, nausea, etc., is retained. The psyche gradually forms out of these already prepared psychic habits which the child holds fast to as a protest against the feeling of being neglected, psychic aptitudes which in the neurosis following a given direction, constitute a symptom picture which may be stated as follows: Act as if you were obliged to shift for yourself by means of one of these faults, of these deficiencies, to gain through it a feeling of superiority. The difference between this and malingering often consists only in this, that in every case it is not always reflection which first calls up the phenomenon, but that the already existing preparedness for the symptom becomes embodied in the web and woof of memory as an insuring agent against the fear of being under-estimated or neglected, just as the technical skill in the fingers of a virtuoso is always ready to respond in the proper reaction to any demand. The whole army of neurotic symptoms, blushing, headache, migraine, fainting, pains, tremor, depression, exaltation, etc., may be traced to these ready-for-use psychic attitudes. One of the facts which, thanks to my method of viewing the subject, I was able to explain concerns the less well known feeling of inferiority common to all girls and women which is due to their feminine rôle in contrast to the masculine. Their soul life is thereby so altered that they constantly betray traits of the "masculine protest" and in truth, usually in a circuitous form, in apparently feminine inferior traits such as are described in the previously cited group. Education as well as the necessary preparations for the future force them to bring their superiority to expression, their "masculine protest" in insidious ways, mostly having the character of resignation. The features of "Emotion" (Heyman's) are always sufficiently distinct, greed for power, envy, desire to please, inclination to cruelty are so apparent that they may be regarded as compensatory masculine traits, as directed towards a masculine goal. Parkes Weber (Lancet, 1911) has, following me, discovered the foundation of hysterical phenomena in this sort of provision against under-estimation.

Preparedness for crime is also to be regarded as an outcome of the masculine protest in persons whose compensatory ideal necessitates a fictitious guiding line which demands that the life, health, and possessions of his fellow man should be stripped of worth. In cases of extreme uncertainty where the deprivations, under-estimations, threaten loss of the feeling of ego-consciousness as well as where there is strained effort to "reach the top," to secure supremacy, such persons (whose feeling of inferiority has sought compensation in emotional preparedness, in essential pursuit of the guiding line, by processes of abstraction from reality) will seek to come nearer to their ideal by a crime. D. A. Jassny has given an excellent analysis of this mechanism which is manifested most clearly in emotional crimes, habitual crimes and crimes of negligence in women, in Gross' Archiv. f. Kriminalanthropologie, 1911.

The great importance of the relations of love in human life has as a result that the neurotic greed to possess everything enters regularly into the relations of man and wife and there develops a disturbing tendency by introducing an inclination to disregard reality and causing the undertaking of enterprises with a view to maximation the feeling of personal worth. It lies in the nature of a neurotic to wish to diminish the feeling of inferiority by constant proofs of his superiority. For this reason, the person loved is forced to sacrifice the personality, to exist entirely through the neurotic who makes this demand, to become a means for augmenting the feeling of personal worth of the neurotic. A good test of a real love without neurotic tendency would be the fact that the person loved was allowed to preserve his or her personal worth or when this personal worth even received support. Such cases are rare. In the relation of the sexes there arises nearly always an obstinate and selfish feature, a tendency to put to test, towards suspicion which constantly disturbs the peaceful marital relations. Arbitrary demands are the order of the day. One situation explains the other, so that the gist of the situation can always be easily recognized. It is as if both parties were confronted by an enigma which they endeavor to solve by every possible means. Analysis always reveals a fear of the sexual partner resulting from a feeling of inferiority and thereby striving toward superiority.

We have already become acquainted to some extent with the strivings by circuitous ways where there is an accentuated feeling of inferiority in congenital defectives. This striving results in a number of neurotically acquired adaptations and certain traits of character assume prominence, so that the individual remains in close touch with the enemy. Perhaps the really most important features are distrust and jealousy, with which desire for mastery and disputatiousness are concurrent. According to the previous history of the patient and to the previous available practices as well as the neurosis which he can apply to his purpose, the one feature or the other declares itself with more or less distinctness. They all stand under the pressure of the fictitious final purpose and break forth when reduction of the feeling of personal worth is threatened, or show that they are still effective when pride represses them into the unconscious. In all cases these individuals have at their disposal the neurotic adaptations, which now in the form of depression, again as anxiety at being left alone, as fear of places, as insomnia, and in a hundred and one other symptoms by means of which they seek to force "the opponent" to lay down his arms. The strongest moral principles have the same value as, for instance, coquetry and adultery as a revenge when the feeling of being under-estimated demands the reinstatement in equality or the gaining of the upper hand of the other party. The husband expresses protesting revengefulness where there is a lack of the feeling of superiority by playing the wild man, in side leaps, in rejection, sometimes however in impotence, in remarkable protection of the children or doubts about their legitimacy, frequently in shunning domesticity, in increased alcoholism or in the pursuit of pleasure. The purpose of this line of conduct is usually so obvious that it is generally understood. For it only then reaches its goal when the wife feels herself thereby degraded. The frequent delirium of jealousy of alcoholics is not based on the resulting impotence, but alcoholism, impotence and the increased jealousy as a trait of character are neurotic forms of expression of those predisposed and whose feeling of inferiority experiences an aggravation. Like all other neurotics such an individual suffers from the neurotic apperception, by means of which he measures the distance of reality from an ideal which has been strengthened in the direction of his tendency. It is, however, one of the most effective attitudes of neurotic individuals to measure *pollice verso* so to speak, real human beings by an ideal, so that their value may be reduced to any desired extent.

The revengefulness of the rejected wife manifests itself preferably in those neurotic symptoms
in which frigidity plays the principal rôle. The
purpose of this is to contest with the husband,
the male force, to show him, even where there is
perfect accord, limits of his power and thus to
secure a considerable superiority.

That this powerful construction is the result of
an original feeling of deficiency which demands
compensation becomes apparent from more thorough analysis. Ordinarily the apperception of
an under-estimation of an analogous fear or of a
wish of this nature takes place after the picture of
the antithesis of "man—woman," in accordance
with which the maximation of the ego-consciousness is felt and valued as "masculine," the lowering as "feminine." Or instead of the feeling of
being under-estimated, in a phantasy or dream of
a castration (feminine) a loss of the penis arises
as a symbol. Very often the masculine guiding
line which had already played an important rôle in
the previous history penetrates into the neurosis
as an essential or accessory component and accentuates the manly traits as soon as the ego-
consciousness enters into the question, a circumstance which as a rule is very striking in women.

Aside from the predisposition to jealousy a
large number of other symptoms are manifested
in female neurotics, which originate from the ad-

herence to the masculine guiding line. These
symptoms usually have reference to love or to the
sexual relation and claim may be made to many
causes as their foundation, instead of the only
right one, the desire to be a man, which as far as
possible seeks realization. This inclination to
love and "manage" then continues throughout
the entire life or this form of the masculine guiding line develops in advanced years an inner contradiction, a fear of not being able to hold the
husband, touches the ego-consciousness and
causes constantly varying neurotic, erotic disturbances. These variations are dependent on
the fact that the new guiding line, to win a husband, in order thereby to elevate the feeling of
personal worth, contains within itself a contradiction: the lowering of the feeling of personality
by assuming the feminine rôle. In such cases
often the neurotic symptom of indecision awakens
and extends to the most banal relations of life,
until the real situation is understood to depend
upon the hermaphroditic attitude of the subject
from which the impulse of indecision and doubt
takes its source. Every decision calls up an antithetical reaction in the opposing consciousness
which is then felt and valued after the antithesis
of "man—woman" so that the patient either simultaneously or in immediate sequence plays a
feminine and then a masculine rôle. The fol-

lowing case may be considered as a visible example of such a condition:

A girl 30 years of age, who earned her living by teaching, complained of uneasiness, constant doubt, insomnia and thoughts of suicide. Since the death of the father she had taken care of the whole family, thus taking the place of the man, the provider, and in her phantasies and dreams is a beast of burden, a horse that must draw all the load. She works until she is exhausted and sacrifices everything to her brother and to her sister. As far back as she can remember, she has always wished she had been a man. As a child, she had sturdy boyish traits and at 15 years of age was still mistaken for a boy at bathing places.

Von Neusser has called attention to these bodily traits of the opposite sex where constitutional anomaly could be shown in his work on the status thymico-lymphaticus. Also in my work on neurology, I have emphasized the finding of bodily traits of the opposite sex and could prove concerning them that they are often made use of by neurotics, either for giving prominence to the inferiority in cases where the femininity is accentuated or for expressing the "masculine protest." The previous observations of Flies who as well as Halvan directed my attention to this field, do not take into consideration the psychic mechanisms as I understand them.

In one variety, this female patient revealed the masculine protest on the very first day by refusing sharp gratuitous treatment. She would receive no t , she repeated emphatically several times in succ ssion and she subsequently explained to me in the manner with which I was already acquainted hat it was unmanly to receive gifts. Therefore she had always refused them. On the other hand, she herself gave willingly, something she often practiced in the family in her rôle of father.

From her history, I emphasize one incident as of importance. An uncle had attempted to violate her in her eighth year. In her terror, she had remained passive, but had never mentioned the attack. After her neurosis had made some progress, she had forced herself to the idea that as a child she was already a sinful creature and capable of yielding to any one, and that she had always remained the same. Thus we have the application of a souvenir for the purpose of reassurance with which we are already acquainted, for the course of this train of thought was that up to her thirtieth year of life she had yielded to all men.

From her tenth year to the twenty-fifth year she asserted that she had practiced masturbation excessively. She developed therefrom a strong feeling of guilt, augmented the conviction of her sinfulness, and arrived at the conclusion that she had rendered herself eternally unworthy to enter into matrimony. This conviction was bound to have an extensive influence on her attitude toward men.

The usual rôle of masturbation in neuroses is as follows, that in consequence thereof, an arrangement of a feeling of guilt arises, but at the same time from the possibility of dispensing with a partner, the feeling of security from being under the influence of a partner. The analogy with those cases where the same security is sought by strengthening the defects of childhood, enuresis, stuttering or other neurotic symptoms is obvious. The original feeling of inferiority remains behind as an echo, fills itself with phantasies of feminine deficiencies and feelings of guilt and forces the individual to strive for the manly guiding point. The conduct of our female patient is constructed according to the guiding line which may be expressed in the words, "I wish to be a man."

A few years ago, a compulsory idea took hold of her which clearly reflects our idea of the neurosis. The patient believed that she had lost through masturbation a part of the genital region which extended forward and which according to her description seemed to her to be a penis. Now she had become wholly unfit for marriage, because she could not live through it if her husband should hear of her sins. The security seems to be thus entirely assured and it is easy to understand how she brings her fictitious masculine guiding principle as an ideal in contrast with her real femininity, emphasizes the latter and feels inferior, yet by this very expedient seeks to exempt herself from a feminine rôle in reality.

But even this assurance, however strong it might seem, became in time insufficient to satisfy the ideal of personal value of our patient. Her female friends deserted her in order to marry, and when finally her younger sister married, her guiding line became no longer tenable because her ambition strove also for "mastery over men." She decided arbitrarily, as nervous girls with extreme indecision usually do, to take the first best. She went to a masquerade where she became acquainted with a worthy man who wished to marry her after a short acquaintance. During a trip she yielded to him because, as she said, she feared that by contact he might become aware of the defect of her genital organs and leave her disgraced and she would rather have anything else happen to her. When later the man in a friendly way insisted on her telling him if he were her first lover and why she had become so cold she threw him overboard with the untruthful explanation that she had had relations with other men. Thereupon the man broke off the affair.

It is easy to imagine what now followed. The patient who was already constantly grieving over another loss than that of her masculinity, beheld herself thwarted and deprived of her new masculine triumph. She recalled her lie which, as she sought to explain to me later, she had told in order to punish the man for having conquered her, in order to deprive him of worth. She explained to him the facts, but he withdrew entirely, for the most part from fear of further discords in a marriage with this neurotic girl. Thereupon our patient became passionately in love with him, made a god of him, passed sleepless nights in thoughts of him, and took an oath to have him or no other husband, for this one was in all human probability lost to her. Thus by means of various expedients of her neurosis she had returned to her original guiding line, and had gained a fictitious ideal and up to the time of her treatment, had succeeded in avoiding the feminine rôle.

In psychotherapeutic treatment, special attention should be given to prevent this blindly working tendency to depreciation of the patient from making the physician himself a victim, as the condition of disease is regularly used as a means of depriving the psycho-therapeutist of his worth. The patient may do this by following the

ordinary direction which his disease takes only
with a sharper tone, because he strengthens the
symptoms, or originates new ones, and tries to
supply tense relations, frequently also situations
of love and friendship, but always with the intention (which is the result of his neurotic tendency,
of the masculine protest) of becoming master of
the physician, of giving him a setback, of making
him play a "feminine" part, of annihilating his
worth. The tactical and pedagogic expedients
to which one is obliged to resort in order to
weaken this struggle of the patient against the
physician, in order to render it comprehensible
and in order to demonstrate in this way the neurotic conduct or attitude of the patient in life
generally, become an important factor in the
therapeusis. The silent protest of the neurotic
should not however be undervalued, and one
should be on the lookout for it to the very end of
the treatment, laying special stress upon it towards its termination. It should be viewed with
quiet, objective composure, as the matter-of-fact
aggressiveness of the patient and as having the
same value as has the neurosis, inasmuch as it
furnishes the neurotic predispositions and traits.
Freud's hypothesis of transference will be referred to again later. It is nothing more than
an expedient of the patient who seeks to rob the
physician of superiority. Bezzola and others

have described the circuitous ways in which the neurotic patient seeks to deprive physicians of their value. It is always the masculine guiding line which is revealed, the purpose of which is to assure the patient's superiority. The most usual manner of enhancing his tendency to aggression, the neurotic finds by holding fast to his symptoms, because these in themselves present a phase of his aggressive tendency.

An extract from a history of a patient shortly before the end of her treatment reveals (in the form of an unfriendly impulse) this effort to deprive the physician of value as a psychic predisposition of her "masculine protest." The patient was placed under treatment because of an anxiety and of crying out at night. She was a virgin, 36 years of age. I will begin the description of this neurotic picture with the following dream:

"I was lying at your feet and reached upward with my hand trying to grasp your clothes which were silk. You made a lascivious gesture, whereupon I said laughingly, 'You are then no better than the other men!' You confirmed this with a nod."

Those who, following Freud's interpretation of dreams, place the sexual wish-motive in the foreground, will not be at a loss for an interpretation; the requirements for a sexual basis for the dream were fully supplied. The requirements could also be complied with, as the patient had already done, by bringing forward a reminiscence from childhood, when she solicited her father in a similar manner; her neurotic tendency to attain security had indeed carefully collected all admonitory experiences, in order to use the man in an "anaphylactic" manner against repetitions. Indeed, one could easily get the assent of the patient to ascribe to repressed impulses of the will the emergence of souvenirs of like tendency and the present experiences. For her neurotic psyche sees such exaggerations as real remembrances and makes them her basis of operation, which she does by affirming her conviction of inferiority, of her fault, of her sin, of her too feminine nature, in order to defend with greater vehemence her superiority, her manliness and to increase her foresight. This increased masculine protest, however, which has its source in the defective perspective of the patient who is overfearful, can not but naturally increase the neurosis. The destruction of this false perspective first (the foundation of the neurotic apperception), and the damming up of the fictitious influx in the direction of the masculine protest, and finally a right understanding of the superstitious faith in an abstract guiding line and the apotheosis of the same are the levers which must be used to remove neurosis.

Our patient had begun a liaison with a married man about the time of this dream. When he pressed himself upon her and invited her to his house during his wife's absence at a watering place, she was troubled with all sorts of scruples, which I strengthened considerably. Nevertheless, she justified the relation and "played with the fire" because she said the impatient writhing of the man amused her. Incidentally, her way of regarding the subject was an inimical act directed against her relatives and against me her monitor. Her own understanding could be interpreted as a reasonable excuse. But the previous history of the patient, and her conduct during her illness which lasted twenty years, and during her treatment, showed plainly that she was strongly under the influence of the masculine protest, and that she could have demanded the subjugation of the man, but that she must have refused to play a feminine rôle—(she suffered from anxiety states and crying out in terror at night). The central point of her psychic attitude consisted in fear of the man to whom she believed she was not equal, a fear which she sought to compensate by her own masculine bearing and by the lower estimation of men.

After this information concerning the patient, we could venture to interpret the dream. She exaggerated her physical dependence on me and gave this conviction form by clothing it in a dream image which is admirably suited for this purpose. "As though I lay at your feet." This being "below" was taken as a basis of operation and we could rightly expect that the manly impetus would follow the construction of a fictitious feminine rôle. She reached upwards with the hands. The contamination contained my deprivation of masculinity. I wore a silk dress. The same psychic mechanism hovers in the remaining part of the dream. I had admonished the patient—in the dream I made a lascivious gesture of which the seducer had been guilty, that is to say that I am on the same level, "I also am not better than the other men." Besides this to carry out the idea further, I was silent and showed assent by a gesture in the dream. The opposite thought that I could be better is insupportable to the patient; from it, which gives me a sort of superiority, originates the preventative dream fiction constructed after the neurotic perspective. The patient only felt secure when all men were alike bad. Then she is following her old guiding line and feels superior. Her superiority is reflected by her laughing in the dream as well as by my silence.

The circumstance that she began this first dangerous liason with a married man is worthy of attention.   In all similar cases, such a relation may be recognized as an effort to obtain security from marriage, usually also from sexual relations.   The masculine guiding line is preserved, but reality asserts itself by feminine excitements and emotions.   It is as I have frequently pointed out, a masculine protest made with feminine means which recalls to me the fact of psychic hermaphroditism.   Finally, too, the superiority over the lawful wife asserts itself in the three-cornered arrangement, something which in all analogous cases strengthens to an unusual degree the motive force.

If we now proceed as it were to a comparative psychology and wish to bring to conscious expression the component parts of the foundation of the apperception of this patient and put the question before us, whence these psychic preparations which lead to the attempt of unmanning the man by feminine means in order to enhance thereby her feeling of worth in a masculine direction and to surpass a woman's, the answer is: From her relation to her father and mother.   There she derived the preparation to approach the father with love and esteem as a guiding ideal, learned to master him and had thus shown herself superior to the mother.   If one abstracts the masculine protest of the neurotic child and if one apperceives these conditions (as neurotics often do) in a sexual scheme the "incest complex" remains. One can now, as I have shown in former works, take out of the incest complex again what the masculine guiding line has placed in it, namely, the assurance of the feeling of personal worth under the title of an amative condition. In the literature on psycho-analysis, the assertion emerges constantly that the libido of the neurotic is fixed on the father or on the mother, on which account he seeks similar amative conditions which are in reality that which was loved in the parents. The "will to power and to seem" constitutes the only amative condition and this guiding point the neurotic seeks with all caution, but invariably, with all his practiced preventive precautions which have originated from and have exclusive value from the craving for security and which resist any change. The significance of the amative feeling is no other than the assurance of the ego-consciousness, and with this the exclusive influence of the same further betrays that the motive force there is to be found in the masculine protest which has already constructed the incest constellation. Where, as in many cases, the attachment to one of the parents is clearly obvious, it is contracted with a purpose,[1] arranged in order to

[1] In accordance with the life-plan, the finale.

escape decisions concerning other partners, to escape marriage. Then usually the neurotic has destroyed the tendency to love and marriage as inconsistent with the masculine final purpose, or has not developed it.

The original of the "three-cornered situation," the incest situation, resolves itself on closer examination into an affair caused by the megalomania of the child who already reveals all of the characteristics of one predisposed to neurosis, i.e., envy, obstinacy, insatiableness, precocity. Without the sexual appetite really taking part therein, thoughts and reflections of the child may come to light which are later valued and represented as sexual when the neurotic tendency to gain security seeks to make such a connection. "I was already as a child, so beyond bounds, so culpable, my sexual appetite was so strong, I have such a criminal tendency, I am so much the slave of love," these are the echoes in the soul of the adult neurotic. "Therefore I must be careful." The impulse to hold to certain appropriate memories, to falsifications of memory, to exaggerating traces of memories arises from a fear of a defeat in life. And where the sexual appetite has really been revealed, where the possibility of incest really existed, the memory is preserved as an admonitory sign. That which diverts the neurotic psyche is not memory or reminiscence, but the

fictitious final purpose which has derived profit-
able situations therefrom.   It is nearly the same
if these reminiscences have been repressed by the
conscious ego, thrust back into the unconscious.
The neurotic character and the other psychic gestures with their unconscious mechanism are none
the less opposed to disposition in proper order in
reality.

Thus it was in the case of our female patient.
She related, for example, that she always wished
to win the father to her side and that she accomplished this by carefully falling in with his train
of thought and his wishes.   It was not difficult to
leave her mother.   From the age of fourteen, she
began to refuse to kiss him because she began to
feel a peculiar erotic emotion.   In explanation of
this, I might add that the patient had from her
twelfth year manifested unmistakable signs of a
neurosis.   Her situation at that time permits us
to understand the significance of this attempt at
security—through the construction of erotic preparations.   She had always been an unruly, boyish creature who had already learned to feel the
force of the sexual appetite and for some time
had already practiced masturbation.   About this
time also, men began to make advances to her to
which she reacted with extreme anxiety.   Her
craving for security had progressed so far that
the patient had strengthened the anxiety prepar-

edness which had been constructed out of real emotions of anxiety which she had originally felt, and now she was able, whenever she feared a defeat in the sense of being obliged to play a feminine rôle, any possible cause of which she was on the alert to anticipate, to develop in a hallucinatory manner, a condition of anxiety, so to speak, discount it, such as would have corresponded for example to the eventuality of pregnancy. This anticipation and hallucinatory awakening of sensations which correspond to a fear of defeat which might arise in the future are the work of the preventive craving for security and constitute, as I have already emphasized,[2] the essential part of hypochondria, of phobia and of numerous neurasthenic and hysterical symptoms. I will only state briefly here that the essential part of a psychosis, too, depends upon a similar dogmatic anticipatory representation of a fear or a wish, which the craving for security offers for the better testimony in a phase of great insecurity, in strong dependence on the fictitious guiding line for the conservation of the ego-consciousness. When our patient foresaw a loss of prestige and provided against it by a condition of anxiety in a hallucinatory manner she felt most secure against it. At times, the hallucinatory emotion needed a further strengthening, then the patient arrived at

[2] "Siphilidophobia," loc. cit.

the compulsory idea that she had killed a new born child. In the analysis this idea in regard to the man, at times a place anxiety, was shown to be connected with an admonition of her mother's. This signifies that the patient rescued from her memories even the words of her mother whom she constantly fought against, in so far as these words were adapted to her tendency to seek security.[3]

Among these preparatory conditions an event occurred which favored greatly the hardy construction of these preparations for security. One of her cousins gave birth to a child out of wedlock, a fact which, in a family of respectable middle class people, caused the greatest excitement, especially as the seducer shook the dust of the place from his feet. Our growing understanding for the development of this girl permits us to understand why this event must have accelerated the development of the neurosis and how it came that the words of the mother to whom she ordinarily showed little attention were given such importance. The patient was from her early childhood wild and boyish and of great strength, preferred boys' games and avoided every feminine emotion. She can still remember with what vehemence she refused to play with dolls or to

[3] Along with this the mother should also be at fault with her apodictic threats.

engage in needlework. The personality of the father preponderated over that of the mother to a remarkable degree. An unmarried aunt who lived with the family of our patient took pleasure in her masculine manners, had a beardlike growth of hair and a masculine voice. To this strong and constantly recurring memory was associated another event of later occurrence and which furnished the necessary resonance to the dominating tendency of the patient to wish to become a man. She remembered that one of her fellow scholars with whom she had long been associated—a pseudo hermaphrodite—was changed into a man. These and similar communications —for example, the special interest for hermaphroditism, are sufficient according to my experience for the preliminary assumption that patients of this sort wish to divest themselves of the appearance of femininity, and wish to assume masculine characteristics, as though they fully believed in the possibility of a metamorphosis and that they invariably make an attempt to push forward to the manly rôle which is considered by them to be the higher. Among these attempts to change fate two interest us particularly—the formation of the neurotic character and the neurotic preparations in the form of the neuroses and their symptoms.

As a trait of character which is not rare with

such patients, I may cite the tendency to expose
nakedness, and indeed in childhood or in later
years, in dreams, in phantasy or in neurotic attacks during which they tear the clothes from the
body as though they would divest themselves of
the modesty which they regard as feminine, as
though they wished to make a parade of fictitious
large masculine genital organs and thus belittle
others.   It may be seen from these cases how one
perversion, that of exhibitionism, does not originate from a congenital sexual constitution, but
that the neurosis which seeks to secure the ego-
consciousness is impelled to suppress the feeling
of inferiority, to overcome it because in this neurosis the lively desire to be a complete man, to be
of great account, finds expression.   The sexual
jargon is there—in merely a form of expression
an "as-if" of the sexual content of the thought
or want, only a symbol of the scheme of life.
Also the feminine, exaggerated modesty of such
patients is an expedient in the opposite direction
for the purpose of deceiving concerning the lack
of masculinity.[4]   The absence of modesty in such
cases answers for the desired masculinity, is the
masculine protest, and more marked immodesty
points invariably to disquieting dreams or
thoughts concerning curtailed genital organs and
hence releases feelings of protest of a masculine

[4] Adler—The masculine attitude in female neurotics, etc.

nature which considerably strengthen the line of ambition, of the desire to be first, to possess everything, of obstinacy.   In the further development of the neurosis the desire for mastery and for conquest as well as the tendency to deprive others of worth may assert itself in the form of castration phantasies and their rationalization (Jones). The inclination to disarm the partner, to constantly feel the assurance of superiority which regularly constitutes the content of exhibitionism are often met with.   At times, the lack of neatness and indecency in girls may be interpreted as a trace of the desire for masculinity.

All of these traits of character although they at times seemed contradictory were all active in one direction toward the fictitious final goal in this patient.   It was not difficult to discover a period of uncertainty in her early childhood as preliminary to her affectation of masculine traits, where she, because of lack of insight, misled by boyish traits and her compensatory ambition, cherished the hope of metamorphosing herself at some future time into a man.   This final purpose of developing from a hermaphroditic condition to a male is easy to perceive if her boyish characteristics are understood as preparations for her fictitious final goal.   Here also belongs her inclination to put on boys' clothes, a phenomenon which as with Hirschfeld's "Transvertiter"

flows from the psychic dynamic just described.
Her ideal was particularly distinct in the phantasies and day dreams of her childhood.   Influenced by fairy stories and myths ("Dwarf Nose,"
"Thousand and One Nights," etc.) she imagined
the most varied changes went on in her, sometimes believed herself changed into a Nix or mer-
maid, in which form a fish tail terminated the
lower parts of the body, which is indicative of
the peculiar sense.   At this time a distinct neurotic symptom set in, in this connection; she could
not walk at times, as if, instead of legs, she had
a fish tail.   Also a shoe fetichism in this connection showed the masculine tendency and developed in the form that she insisted on wearing
large shoes, we might say masculine shoes, because her feet hurt.   From Ovid's Metamorphosis which in her rage for reading soon fell into
her hands, she borrowed another fiction which
emerged during her treatment in her dreams; she
imagined she had been metamorphosed in such a
way that the lower part of her body became a
firmly rooted trunk.   In this and in similar ways,
she gave to herself the answer to the question
concerning her future sexual rôle.

We will not be surprised to find that in this and
similar cases, the attitude towards woman was
also influenced by the masculine final goal.   In
the preparations for the future the amative and

sexual relations must have had a place and there-fore we soon find our patient assuming the ideal masculine rôle of protector to a younger and weaker sister. Furthermore, there were sadistic acts towards little girls and servants, but also towards little, girlish boys. Thus we find in the masculine guiding line of the patient an intermix-ture of secondary features, auxiliary traits of homosexuality [5] and masculine sadism, whose ar-rangement resulted from the construction of the masculine predispositions and which is the only possible substitute if masculine sexuality were se-lected by her neurotic apperception from the im-pressions of life. As will be shown, both of these perversions are circuitous ways and expedients, secondary guiding lines which grow out of the ex-aggerated masculine protest. The question con-cerning a constitutional tendency to perversions is wholly irrelevant, because the neurosis seeking assurance and choosing its material in conform-ity with this tendency can fasten upon the most harmless relations, lend to them proportions and value which may become immeasurable in so far as the neurosis requires this by exaggerating them and lending them high values.

[5] Moll has emphasized sharply the frequent association of homo-sexuality with exhibitionism. Our discussion reveals the inner re-lationship. Both perverse tendencies are expressions of the mas-culine protest.

One day as the patient, now fourteen years of age, was accosted by a man on the stairs who made advances to her, an insane idea developed on this foundation which is easy to see through. She imagined herself for many months the murderer of domestic servants (Hugo Schenk) and thus by means of extreme abstractions which were introduced for the purpose of security, she effected an interlacing of her masculine, her homosexual and her sadistic fiction, while she brought them to more distinct expression and at the same time held herself in anticipation of an event which she feared. These three conditions, mere abstractions from reality, strengthening of guiding lines leading to masculinity and upwards, and anticipation of the directing ideal mostly in a disguised form, are the fundamental components of the psychotic construction. The rôle of indigenous and exogenous poisons consists in many cases in the circumstance that these call up a feeling of heightened insecurity which can also result from psychic experiences. But the neurotic tendency toward security, which is strengthened in cases of increased uncertainty, is always the effective cause of the psychotic construction. It then draws more forcibly into its power the neurotic method of apperception and thus causes a "barring off" (*absperrung*). The use of female domestic servants in the psychic construction of our patient brings to expression the tendency to depreciation of females.   In her insane system anxiety is strongly manifested and is distinctly recognizable as a means to obtain security against the male and thus coördinated to the purpose of her insanity constituting a second expression of her aggravated masculine protest.[6]

A further perversion of our patient of which she was dimly conscious consisted in a fellatio phantasy.   The realities connected therewith and which found application in the neurotic tendency of her phantasy were well known to the patient. She had always been very dainty and as a child had always been a slave to this tendency.   Even to-day this characteristic often asserts itself. But it happened not infrequently that she took loathsome things into her mouth without disgust. In her avoidance of the feminine rôle this patient tried, because parturition seemed to her unacceptable and especially feminine, to imagine this perverse situation temporarily possible. The suggestion originated from a conversation which she had overheard.   This perversion was

[6] The accentuation of the fictitious guiding line in the neurotic who becomes insecure is responsible for the fact that he has to utilize stronger measures for the purpose of gaining security. Anxiety where another merely visualizes, hypochondriasis where another employs caution. Our patient had both the anxiety and the delusion where for other girls morality and caution were still sufficient. Thus also in place of caution, hallucinations, and fears.

asserted of a female neighbor living independently and in pleasant relations. Early forced away from the partner, she nevertheless sought to keep in touch with reality and found in the avoidance of labor, supported by her exaggerated leaning to disgusting procedures the way to this, perverse phantasy. But her masculine protest opposed even this. Her crying out at night was as a rule over dream situations of this sort, arranged tentatively, and with this masculine protest, she answered to the femininely perverse rôle which she imputed to herself.

The psychic attitude of the patient described at the beginning shows the essential difference. At least a part of her fear of the man and of the masculine protest was present which after a short time made room for a normal attitude. What could make one apprehensive was the disposition to a difficult, socially inferior situation which could only be obviated by further inroads. Could there, however, be expected a much more favorable solution of the problem of this patient who has declined and who has been robbed of all social connections by the long duration of the neurosis, and is destitute?

With all the solidity and obstinacy which cling to neurotic symptoms and the neurotic character there is often a changeableness and instability which has attracted the attention of many writers. The character of capriciousness, of uncertainty of temper, of suggestibility and of susceptibility to influence (Janet, Strümpell, Raimann and others) was wrongly given as an important sign of a psychogenic affection. But attention must, however, be called to the fact that in psychic phenomena which, as we have shown, only present means, modes of expression and purposeful dispositions, variability must often be preserved among the other characteristics, because it may also occur as an auxiliary line and serve the fictitious final goal, the maximating of the ego-consciousness. The neurotic self-valuation will at any rate take those variations as a point of departure for a way of thinking, will exaggerate the judgment of weakness by strengthening the suggestibility, will support it with selected neuroses for the most part falsely estimated in order to gain in a neurosis a strengthened impetus. As the following case teaches for example. A short time ago, a Viennese physician brought forward in a public session, examples of making waking suggestions which indeed succeeded with a certain lady on a few evenings. When the same lady was expected to offer herself again for a demonstration on a subsequent evening she responded with an hysterical attack of such nature that the further demonstrations were forbidden by the police. In the psychotherapeutic treatment, one must always be prepared for the circumstance that the introduction of the patient into the experiment heightens the masculine protest and the disposition to attacks and is above all forced to prevent this reaction. Every improvement in the condition is felt by the patient as compulsion and conquest and a relapse often follows from no other reason than that an improvement had preceded. The many ambivalent traits of neurotics and psychotic patients arranged according to a polar principle (Bleuler) are constructed on the hermaphroditic splitting of the neurotic psyche and obey exclusively the ideal of personal worth reassured by hypersensibility and great caution.

CHAPTER III

NEUROTIC PRINCIPLES: SYMPATHY, COQUETRY, NARCISSISM, PSYCHIC HERMAPHRODITISM, HALLUCINATORY SECURITY, VIRTUE, CONSCIENCE, PEDANTRY, FANATIC ATTACHMENT TO TRUTH

IN our preceding observation we were able to follow the various attempts, preparations and dispositions of a patient which were conditioned by the setting in of the masculine tendency. The resulting fear of the man was so great that every amative relation was prevented until treatment made it possible. In very many cases the masculine protest manifests itself in an apparently opposite direction. The patients constantly begin new relations which, however, easily languish and are menaced by peculiar turns of fortune. On the other hand, they are capable of contracting marriage one or more times and also of dissolving the marriage again. Very often the deepest passions of love are shown which are strong enough to overcome all obstacles and are usually only augmented by them. The same phenomeha are observed in male neurotics. Upon closer obser-

vation the well known traits of the neurotic subject are again found (first of all the desire for
mastery) which make use of the relations of life
as a vehicle for realizing themselves demonstrably
in the same manner as do his other characteristics.
The desire to possess everything finds expression
in such a way that all men, at times, all human
beings, become an object for conquest and in pursuing this object, coquetry, necessity for tenderness, and discontent with the lot assigned by fate,
play an important part. The preference for
difficulties is often remarkable. A little girl prefers only big men, or love first declares itself when
the parents forbid it, while the attainable is
treated with open disdain. In the conversation
and deliberation of such girls the limiting word
emerges constantly. They wish only a cultured,
only a broad, only a masculine man, only a platonic love, only a marriage without children, only
a husband who will permit their entire liberty, etc.
The tendency toward detraction is often so obvious in this process that hardly a man remains who
would fit the requirements. Usually they have
a completed, often unconscious ideal, in whom
are mingled the features of the father, the
brother, an imaginary personage, or a literary or
historical character. The more we become acquainted with these ideals, the more are we convinced that they are advanced as a fictitious

standard in order to detract from reality by comparison with them. The psychic tendency with the accompanying features of an "unwomanly" nature, which frequently gives rise to sexual liberty, unfaithfulness and unchastity, reveals obviously a striving after the masculine ideal. Analysis often shows original organic inferiority, an exaggerated feeling of inferiority, a remarkable original higher estimation of the male which follows on the heels of detraction as a means of assurance. Other assurances strengthen the opinion we have formed. Such ideas as, all men are rough, tyrannical, have a bad odor, are infected, etc., reveal the influence upon apperception of this trend. In male neurotics are observed ideas of a suspicious nature which make the accusation that all women are sinful, unstable, frivolous, psychologically weak-minded, abandoned unrestrainedly to their sexuality.

Our teachers, philosophers and poets, who form the ideal of our time, the Secret Emperor ("heimlichen Kaiser") (Simmel), are also not infrequently under the sway of the same fictions. The neurotic is therefore likely to seize upon them in order to gain a firm guiding line in the unrest of life. For the above neurotic tendency, Schopenhauer, Strindberg, Moebius, and Weininger, besides the religious teachers and fathers of the church, have produced the most pleasing *cleichè.* The *malleus malificarium* and the disgrace of the burning of witches followed the learned disputes of the clerics over the question whether woman has a soul, whether she is a human being. The reassuring schematic fictions of neurotic girls are derived from a childish view of the world because art is still, nearly exclusively, masculine territory and the apperception offers a material less suited to it, and therefore these fictions of neurotic girls are brought into harmony with reality with greater difficulty.

Where reality, however, is able to influence the neurotic fiction of the girl it usually causes traits of character and tendencies which reveal clearly enough the masculine inclination to conquer man, or where there is the strongest tendency to gain security—in a homosexual way—to conquer woman, but which make these neurotics nevertheless seek, as a lover or as a husband, the man to whom she denies value and who is only fitted in a small degree for conflict. The expression of sympathy can in such cases often disguise the state of affairs, and love is then free if the man is powerless, enfeebled, a cripple, aged. In phantasies, dreams and hallucinations in which the man is castrated or changed into a woman, or corpse, is "below," and especially in the tendency to see the man without weapons, small, abased; is revealed the compulsion of the masculine guiding fiction and finds in necrophilia its highest expression.[1]   Another road, as we have already stated, leads over the line of the desire to possess everything, towards neurotic coquetry. The masculine protest is therein revealed, first in the tendency to compensate a feeling of inferiority, of deficiency apperceived through the picture of the lost masculine member by means of domination of many or of all men.   Secondly, by the refusal of a feminine rôle in sexual relations, in marriage.   In place of this despised rôle, expedients are resorted to which are dictated by the manly guiding line, such as sexual anesthesia and perversions of all sorts, among which the sadistic predominates.   Bloch has emphasized in a fine manner the desire for domination by the coquette when he says: ("Beitrage zur Ätiologie der Psychopathia sex," 1903) "Coquetry, which may be defined as the effort of women to attach men to them, makes use, to a considerable extent, of purely sexual means to attain its object, and is, in this respect, an efflux of the true gynecokratic instinct."   We can only add that these "gynecokratic instincts" are constructed according to the picture of the resemblance to men and thus prove themselves to be dependent on a masculine ideal although in the

[1] Eulenburg emphasized in the same manner the relationship between active algolagnia (v. Schrenck-Notzing) and necrophilia.

attainment thereof feminine means are resorted to as expedients because they are the only ones at hand. The attention and interest of these neurotics (among whom the masculine coquettes are remarkable because they seek to carry through their triumph valued as masculine by feminine means) is directed towards making an impression and to force others into their service. A result of this trait of character is that the neurotic strengthening of these secondary guiding lines leads to overestimation of self and therefore also to exaggeration of the desire for mastery, of pride, and of the tendency to detract from the worth of others. Hence we need not be surprised that the object of the desire, as a rule, appears to be overvalued through the narcissism (Naecke) of the patient. This overestimation is rather an *a priori* condition in the construction of the relation and in it is reflected the exaggerated ego of the female patient.[2]

In the psychotherapeutic treatment these cases produce especially the appearance of "being in love with the physician." It may, however, be easily seen that this "transfer of love" corresponds to one of the numerous preparations for conflict used for overcoming the obstacle and thus to get the better of the superiority of the

[2] The belief in personal magic is so strong that every resistance leads to new endeavors.

man, of the masculine physician; and it may be easily seen that the feeling of deficiency which calls forth this peculiar obscure form of the masculine protest springs from their femininity which they feel as inferiority. In no case, however, no matter how far the neurotic may carry coquetry, does it reach far enough to include subjection to the man. Sooner or later the man is threatened with defeat which carries with it loss of dignity, and in fact, always when the neurotic patient feels the situation to be too feminine. This moment may arrive at different stages but it is as a rule, contact, a kiss, expectation of sexual relations, fear of pregnancy or of childbirth which releases the heightened tendency to gain reassurance and causes the outbreak of that which is ordinarily termed a neurosis or psychosis. Then the stronger abstraction of reality comes into its right, the fictions assert themselves with greater distinctness, the tendency to detract from the value of the man leads to actions and deeds which apparently have lost all meaning, and the inimical dispositions of the aggressiveness, and with these the neurotic traits of character come to light.

Every neurotic possesses to some degree this coquetry which has its origin in narcissism. They originate indeed from his hypostasized idea of personal value and is founded like this upon an original feeling of inferiority. The fact that neurotics, especially the species just described, find it so hard to separate themselves from persons or things is in harmony with this. The parting from a person, seemingly not in close relations with the neurotic, to say nothing of a seemingly loved person, is capable of producing the most severe neurotic symptoms, neuralgic attacks, depression, loss of sleep, attacks of weeping, etc. On the other hand, threats of desertion or separation are not rare and are used to bring forth proof of the influence over the person threatened. That the masculine protest is dominant in this coquetry is proved from various phenomena. The strong disinclination for a distinctly feminine rôle has already been emphasized; it is capable in these cases of calling forth a remarkable picture, the appearance of a double life—a splitting of consciousness, an ambivalence (Bleuler). Analysis constantly furnishes greater proof for the striving toward masculinity. Dreams, phantasies, hallucinations, onset of psychosis show in a most distinct manner the striving to become a man, or one of the equivalents, as fear of a feminine lot. The strong tendency toward detraction of men originates from the effort to attain an equal value with the male and gives rise in sexual events to the masculine rôle, which is revealed in frigidity, in desire to be first and in those perversions which force the man to take a slavish and debasing position.

Often the onset of the neurosis may be assumed to have set in when such symptoms as fear of a decision, of a test, of marriage, public appearance, of place (Platzangst), require medical treatment. These anxieties arise at the emerging of a contradiction in the masculine protest, if in pursuing the same a set-back, a feminine lot, a defeat is threatened and hence the forced admission of femininity.

This was the case with one of my patients who, several years ago, just before her first public appearance, became ill with piano-player's cramp. This neurosis furnished a good excuse for escaping from a dreaded failure. The closer examination into the conditions of this illness showed a neurotic illusion in which the patient at the sight of notes was reminded of male genital organs. The first explanation to suggest itself was that of an exaggerated or repressed sexuality whose reflection in the piano-player's cramp was to be sought in the repression of the inclination to masturbation. The result furnished an entirely different explanation. The triumph before the public was supposed to signify an equality with the man, masculinity. This fiction was in contradiction with reality, with her femininity, so that a public appearance equaled a final balancing of the facts (many talented girls and women are wrecked for the same reason). The sense of reality of the patient placed instead of the facts would not admit this condition of things, and arranged by a symbolic interpretation of the heads of the notes works a fictitious abstraction which recalled the femininity and became a regressive signal. The contradiction in the masculine protest of this patient is manifested, as is nearly always the case in the neurosis, in the unrealizability of the fiction just when before the decision the possibility of a failure estimated as "feminine" in character emerged —a common phenomenon which needs no explanation. Now the traits of anxiety, of shyness, of stage-fright are strengthened and they either themselves furnish excuses or preparations and predispositions (in our case pains and inability to move the hands) and divert the attention from the menace to the masculine protest. But in this case also the force of the masculine protest is astonishing, it forms a preparedness for conflict in the direction of the masculine protest even out of the illness in which the patient takes refuge. This girl had entered upon the career of a virtuoso against her will, forced thereto by her unyielding mother. The wrecking of her mother's ambitious plans meant for the daughter a

victory which recompensed her in part. That
which her obstinacy, her masculine tendency was
not able to accomplish, was successful through
her illness as soon as note-stems called up to her
the menacing souvenir "you are a woman, take
care, do not allow yourself to be forced to a feminine obedient rôle by your mother—conquer her."
A further construction, an excuse which yielded
a foundation for the attitude toward her mother,
lay in the heightened feeling that her younger
sister was given preference. This train of
thought, as well as her efforts to gain exclusive
control over every one, her mother, all the members of the family, all human beings in the environment, even of a dog, was reflected in the
heightened characteristics of her coquetry and
found expression, for example, in one of her
latest dreams concerning the physician. The
dream was as follows:

*"I sit opposite you and ask if you like all the
patients as well as you like me. You answered,
'Yes, all, and my four children, too.' All at once
you changed into a woman and went to sleep. A
woman was looking at the black notes."*

The amative disposition of this patient could
endure no rival. She made use of the certainty
of her conquest in order to support her feeling
of security. The physician who gave her to un-

derstand that he treated all patients with the same interest, and who loved his children besides, becomes forthwith the point of attack of her striving for domination, as was formerly the mother, the man whom she married, as were all persons in her environment, domestic servants, trades-people, teachers, etc. Her self-centered nature did not need to "transfer," as she came to the treatment with rigid predispositions and put them in play from the first moment of her meeting with the physician. Only the new situation was surrounded with difficulties and obstacles which prevented the will to domination through love from fully developing. Naturally my wife was left out of the dream. Just this omission is the cornerstone of the situation; my wife is definitely set aside. Up to this point the feminine means extend and characterize the feminine line to which the patient holds. Now the masculine protest emerges more distinctly. I become unmanned, the reassuring illusion of the patient, namely, the notes as a protecting symbol of the male genitals, asserts its right. She, herself, "takes care," secures herself in order not to sink in her feeling of masculine ego-consciousness, to suffer no defeat.

That I go to sleep in the dream, assigns to me a place similar to that which her husband occupies. The patient feels it as a great neglect that

her husband, an overworked manufacturer, often
goes to sleep before she does. The unmanning
of the husband is the answer thereto, as well as
a prolonged insomnia whose constructive significance lies in the fact that it permits the patient
to operate against her husband. Now she could
refuse him his right as a husband and turned him,
at first in the middle of the night, later permanently, out of her bedroom; because he "snored
and disturbed her so much." Our patient would
have easily found another argument if this one
had not presented itself, and it would be erroneous to exclude the neurotic construction as a
cause because in this case the neurotic happened
to be right. In order to prove that she is right
the patient will often argue aptly; the neurotic
stigma in fact consists in the tendency to render
the superiority visible by all possible means.
Litigious paranoia for example reveals this
mechanism to us with greater clearness. Besides, the neurosis of our patient continues in its
construction of assurances. To her insomnia is
added, in order to place this on a firmer basis, a
sensitiveness of hearing, whose mechanism consists in an overcharging of the attention for the
purpose of serving the neurotic tendency, so that
we were also able to say, by this overcharging,
the patient is awakened by the slightest noise as
soon as she falls asleep. Thus she can, still awake

when morning comes, sleep far into the day and thus avoid the feminine tasks of the household, in the same manner as she had escaped the mother's domination by stage fright and cramps in the fingers. An auditory hallucination, a sawing noise, constitutes a final security which may be pursued analytically in two directions. The one interpretation is furnished by a warning souvenir which at the same time is an incentive to her coquetry—once, when eight years old, she overheard an intimate scene at her married sister's, she felt shut out, neglected—she gave a similar value to her husband's "indifference" when he fell asleep before she did, in order to be able to take a sharply aggressive attitude toward him. A second interpretation led in another direction. The noise recalled the sawing off of a stem and symbolized, acoustically,[3] the unmanning, the detraction from the worth of the man. As is also so frequently the case this symptom proved to be (just as I have maintained of the dream, of symptoms, and of the neurosis) a representative instance of the ascension from the feminine to the masculine line, as a masculine protest against a situation usually previously felt as feminine,

[3] One is reminded here of the somatic-jargon of which we have already spoken. Thus the words, "schrill" and "grell," bring to expression sensorially in their transformed meaning, analogies which are felt at one time through the eye, at another, through the ear.

against an anticipated feeling of defeat and as a symbol of the life scheme of this neurotic patient.

This, and similar cases, explained to me in what manner suggestibility became an auxiliary of the tendency to attain security, either because therefrom the patient gained in small things the conviction of her weakness in order to provide herself with proper protection at critical times, or because the patient yields with surprising pliability in order to gain ascendancy over the other person.[4] The more direct efforts of her tendency to domination stand so sharply in contrast with this yielding that when only superficially observed the phenomenon resembles a splitting of consciousness. In the same manner, vanity, pride, and self-admiration will guide the patient in many cases to the same goal, while she at times, conducts herself with modesty, simplicity, and carelessness, using these qualities as expedients. Usually externals and attitudes are carefully studied. Very often fetichism is manifested, whose essential and constructive foundation represents efforts to prove equality with men in circuitous ways, hence to compensate for a feeling of deficiency. Literature furnishes us

[4] The latter mechanism seems to be at the root of passive homosexuality while both attitudes may be taken as the structure of masochism, still better, pseudomasochism.

with representations of all these efforts in a most refined form in the memoirs of Baschkirzewa and Helen Rakowiza. Analyses of a series of cases where the memories of these remarkable impressions from childhood had been preserved more vividly than usual furnished me with interesting verifications at a time when I was already far advanced in my exposition of the doubts about the future sexual rôle on the part of the neurotic child and the masculine protest which necessarily springs therefrom. Some remembered very distinctly having been in doubt up to the twelfth or thirteenth year whether they were male or female. It may not be a matter of chance that these were male patients. At times the doubt emerged whether they were not hermaphrodites, so that I am inclined to think that in other cases where the thought of hermaphrodites was distinctly and importunately present in the memory of the patient and was spontaneously brought forward, it is the last impression of a doubt about the patient's own sex. And in literature, too, I have frequently run across this significant trace in the histories of neurotics and psychotics without the significance of this doubt concerning the sexual rôle being clear to the writers. Meschede described an interesting case of question-compulsion (Fragezwang), and Freud one of dementia after Schreber's biography. I disregard whether or not this interest of the patient was explained by illustrations, or placards, in the lexicon, by readings by spectacles, by occurrences, as well as the scientific interpretation which seemed to concentrate its attention to the male periods, the male climacteric, to the examination of the male or female share in the individual, etc. For me, the permanent impression which asserted itself in an obvious emphasis of the relation and the reciprocal relation of the antithesis male-female, was the important factor.

In recent years since I have hit upon these fundamental phenomena of the neurosis, I have often asked myself if I, too, in the course of my development from childhood was not dominated by a similar doubt notwithstanding the fact that the question of hermaphroditism only attracted me at a very late period and from the standpoint of a critic, and hence in a secondary manner. Also my rejection of the biological hermaphroditism as a cause of the neurosis (Flies) I would use as an argument against such doubts in my early youth, if I were not familiar with the fact that often the negation is the assertion of an old interest which has become unconscious. But my view of life shows me that I must have become master of old childish contrary tendencies, without the exaggerated masculine protest having been developed. Because I have in life, as well as in science, after a first abstract valuation of the masculine principle over the feminine, rejected the flood of arguments to prove the original deficiencies of women, with pertinent calmness.

I believe, however, concerning the former critics of the "masculine protest," from the manner in which they have undertaken the contest, and from their stubborn failure to understand it, that the exaggerated savageness of their attack in a strictly scientific question is referable nearly as much as is their fear of the concept "hermaphroditism" to a childhood impression which alarmingly presented to them an accentuated effeminacy or hermaphroditism, with which, however, it is not my intention to deter any one from a scientific criticism.

Besides, there is no better way of judging the reaction of the neurotic psyche than from the answers to questions showing estimation of the opposite sex. It will become apparent that every stronger denial of the equality of the sexes, every detraction or overvaluation of the opposite sex is invariably connected with a neurotic disposition and neurotic traits. They are all dependent on the neurotic tendency to obtain security, and all manifest distinct traces of the masculine protest and are evidence of the essential, more abstract adherence to a guiding fiction.

They are one and all, expedients of human thought to enhance the feeling of personal worth.

It follows from the exposition of my psychology of the neuroses that children with male as well as those with female tendencies, look forward with fear to the lot of a woman, to be subject to a man, to be deprived of virginity, injured, to be obliged to bear children, to play a subordinate rôle in life, to obey, to be backward in knowledge, in skill, in strength, wisdom, to be weak, to have periods, to become a sacrifice to husband and children, to become at last an old and neglected woman. How this fear of the future gives rise to egoistic traits of character has been described above. I have described a typical case of a little girl in the "Disposition zur Neurose" (l. c.).

I am able to show in the case of a patient suffering from a gastric neurosis a line of conduct which is regularly observed in the psychic development of neurotic patients. This is the anticipation in thought and emotion of all disadvantages which could be expected to occur. This tendency is observed in early childhood when, where there is organic inferiority and the evils arising therefrom, it is of excessive growth. Very often this feeling occurs at the time immediately preceding the falling asleep and it is then not remarkable that a dream fiction spurs further this effort of anticipation in a form to cause fear. Only the dream, in resemblance to the hallucination, brings with it a condition of feeling, of emotion, which has the significance as anticipation of emotion parallel to anticipation in thought in a waking condition. The hallucinatory excitability is, as I have already emphasized in the "Studie über Mindwertigkeit von Organ," an extended capacity of the brain which is overstrained in compensatory directions, serves the neurotic tendency to gain security and owes its representative faculty in consciousness to the memory which follows a certain tendency to the neurotic, cautious apperception. The childish undeveloped psyche shows at most, traces of tendencies toward hallucinatory feelings which are to be understood as the fictitious preparations for a goal, as anticipation in time of uncertainty.

Thus laughing in sleep, or pleasant sensations in the anticipatory quest of organic satisfaction, or of security. The hallucinatory excitement in the neuroses and psychoses always, and without exception, serves the guiding fiction of the ideal of personality. The significance of the hallucinations of pain and anxiety for the fiction of nervous diseases should also be taken into account. A further examination of the mechanism of the hallucination teaches us unequivocally that it is composed of tendencies to abstraction and to anticipation, and that it gains significance as a strengthened fiction or as a warning souvenir because it acts as a spur to the assurance of the feeling of personal worth. That they are connected with traces of memory has no essential significance. The psyche works without exception with the content of consciousness and with sensations that are given by experience and originate in the corporal substratum. The significance of the psyche, and especially of the neurotic psyche, lies in the special choice of these memory traces and in their connection with the neurotic apperception which gives them their trend. Therefore the nervously exalted tendency to gain security makes use of a specially developed function of prevision, of hallucination, in which abstractly and imaginatively a scene unrolls, an anticipated dénouement, a foreseen finale, with eagerness so that the hallucinated individual builds the bridges to it, or they have an admonitory quality warning them to choose another way. Hallucinations as well as dreams are, like other tentatives of the psyche, fitted for finding the way which leads to the maximation or preservation of the ego-consciousness. In it are reflected the faiths, the hopes or the fears of the patient.

The above patient was on the eve of marriage when her gastric neurosis began. She suffered from pains in the region of the stomach, belching, vomiting, loss of appetite and obstipation. One evening, shortly before going to sleep she heard the word "Eskadambra" distinctly. The formation of apparently meaningless words are often among the performances of neurotics. Usually they prove to be put together according to a plan, just as children invent languages by means of which they attain a feeling of superiority. Pfister was able to make interpretations of the word pictures which originated from fascination in the cases of those having the "gift of tongues."

In a previous chapter I have given a solution of an hallucinatory "sawing" in the ears, in two other cases I found the roaring serving as an admonitory memory on the roaring of the sea and its dangers as a sense-picture of life, just as Homer compares the ἀγορὰ to the roaring sea.[5]

In paranoia and dementia præcox the emotions leading to the masculine protest disguise themselves in the form of hallucinations and assure the psychotic scheme through their acoustic or visual complement. Likewise concerning the above mentioned rounding off of a psychic move into a hallucination of hearing, we may assume

[5] On another occasion I found roaring in the ears to be a reminder of the tones of telegraph wires. These tones reminded him of his isolation in childhood where alone he often embraced the world as does the telegraph, with his hopes for the future.

that a strong inner necessity has led to a greater tension of the tendency to gain security, for which the word "eskadambra" though without value or significance for the patient, can represent a signal or sign.[6]   One is justified in thinking, however, that a thorough understanding of this word would show a meaning which would reveal to us the mental condition of this girl.   As a rule it is easy to obtain an understanding of hallucinations of this sort, at least not more difficult than for short fragments of dreams.   Asked concerning the impression of the new-word formation, the patient answered, she recalled "alhambra" by this word.   For this she had evidently always had a great interest; once it stood proudly, but it was now fallen into decay, a ruin. The beginning of the word "Esk" was to be found in the word "Eskimo," in "E(tru)skan" too, these letters are found.   The race of "Baskes" occurred also to her; in this word the greater part of "Esk" appears.   The patient thus indicates the way she has followed in the construction of the new word, she has joined a fragment of the names of ancient tribes and the name of a ruined city.   Finally the word "alhambra" had for her also only the significance

[6] As one has to assume also concerning the dream which represents the image of a psychic movement in the state of consciousness.

of a fragment, and hence we are justified in assuming the thought of being broken, made small, made short, would emerge in the interpretation of the hallucination. The letters "skad" belong, as the patient easily discovered, to the word "kaskade." She said she was certain of this because she had used the expression "ganze kaskaden" in connection with the period, the menstrual period just passed.

When it is taken into consideration that this patient was about to be married the connection of this construction of new words with the psychic condition can be understood without anything further. That she is disinclined to marry one can see from her neurosis, which formed a ready obstacle.[7] In the hallucination there is a disconnected sketch of the following train of thought: the glory of my virginity will be destroyed—I shall bear a new race—I will be forced to sacrifice whole cascades of blood. When I had brought the interpretation up to this point, the patient helped me further by relating that when she was eight years old she had heard that a woman of her acquaintance had died from loss of blood at the birth of a child. Since then she

[7] As has already been mentioned, the anticipation of marriage furnishes one of the most potent moments for the accentuation of a neurosis or for the development of a psychosis. The contrary expressions of these patients, such, for instance, as "I would very much like to be married," always prove themselves to be platonic.

had always been afraid of childbirth. What now is the meaning of this hallucination? Can it be defined, even remotely, by the word "wish-fulfillment"? The meaning of this new formation of words is the anticipatory interpretation in the direction of a danger to be feared, of being humiliated, or the fear of becoming a ruin, as she had often called her mother, of dying like the woman she remembered in her childhood. This feeling against female functions (and the patient indeed strove also consciously against marriage) is of older date, originated in early childhood, and was at that time embodied in the wish to be ahead, healthy, strong like her father. It became then a fictitious guiding line and was filled with a logical content, which was grouped about a masculine ideal of personality, and was filled also with a fear in the same direction against a feminine rôle. Now I was able also to make clear to the patient the meaning of her stomach neurosis. It was a hallucinatory excitement which reflected the hardships of pregnancy, warning the patient to avoid the same. In the waking condition, in the dream and in hallucinations and in the neurosis there was a harmony of the tendency towards security—do not be a woman, do not submit, be a man!

This girl manifested in her demeanor rough, resolute traits, and could get along with no one.

Her ambition flamed blazingly and made her intolerant. She required unconditional submission from her fiancé whom she treated very badly and with whom she often dissolved all relations. Once, however, when he turned his attention to another girl, she offered everything in order to hold him. One of the day dreams of her childhood consisted in the phantasy that the whole human race was going to destruction and that she alone would remain, an analogy with the myth of the flood in which the ego-centric, inimical nature of the patient is clearly manifested.

In the cases of many patients who show signs of the tendency to "have everything" as in the case of the girl just described, traits of character of an opposite nature are found. They are often of such importunate honorableness, modesty and contentedness that the peculiar accentuation of these qualities awakens the suspicion of a special arrangement. Their conscience always makes itself heard and their feeling of being at fault is always ready to react on the slightest occasion.[8]

The solution of this enigma which has puzzled humanity for a long time, is furnished by an understanding of the craving for security which breaks through the direct aggressive guiding line, and which puts an end to greed and immod-

[8] Adler, "Ueber neurotische Disposition," l. c., and Fortmül-ler, l. c.

eration as soon as the egoistic ideal is threatened by them. Conscience then constitutes, so to speak, an intermediate guiding fiction, as does also its anticipatory exaltation, the abstract self-accusation of guilt. These are instances in which all actions planned and anticipatory preparations are changed around in such a way that they are not injurious, that they permit the feeling of personal worth to be preserved. We perceive on this point the opposition in the original feeling of inferiority as a compensation for the feeling of uncertainty which has come to moral expression. Now the neurotic can exclude a number of possibilities which could degrade him. In other relations, also, the effect of the craving for security is recognizable, in morals, in religion, in superstition, in stirrings of conscience and in the feeling of guilt. They all form themselves into rigid formulæ and principles such as the uncertain neurotic loves. And he can prepare himself by practice in small things, test his moral strength on mere nothings and especially—*principiis obsta!*—secures himself from a moral fall which he exaggerates in anticipation by feeling the moral defeat beforehand. This last hallucinatory expedient resembles the security through neurotic anxiety, and indeed conscientiousness, self-accusation, and anxiety often complement each other, or alternate with each other, in the neurosis. The knowledge of this fact is of great importance to the psycho-therapeutist for the understanding of the connection between masturbation and neurosis and from which may be comprehended the significance as a security of the feeling of self-accusation constructed from the fact of onanism. If this feeling of guilt is brought into junction with the masturbation for the purpose of working as a brake against the force of sexuality, both constitute, later, a base of operation from which the patient augments his neurotic disposition in order to guard against a reduction of his ego-consciousness. As a rule, both—with the assistance of anticipated results, as impotence, tabes, paralysis, loss of memory—are used as an excuse in order to avoid making decisions, and always also for deepening the fear of the sexual partner. I have often described connections of this sort in this and in previous works. In the neurosis, honorableness and conscientiousness border on pedantry, therefore we will not be surprised to find how often these qualities draw their real value from the fact that thereby the neurotic is placed in a position to humiliate others, to come into conflict with them, to raise himself above others and press them into his service. It is just the neurotic whose tendency to dominate contains the scheme "to possess everything" and who not rarely preserves mem-

ories of sins, who will usually take care not to
betray a secret which would certainly result in
his humiliation. He will rather seek to preserve
the appearance even with great pains and anxiety; will blush anxiously when he lifts his own
pocketbook from the floor, and will avoid being
alone in a strange room in order not to fall under
suspicion of theft, if something should be missed.
In like manner I found an obstinate wish to pay
in advance, to owe nothing, in patients to whom
every expenditure seemed a reduction of their
ego-consciousness. They preferred undergoing
an evil and making an end of it to enduring one
without end, but had at the same time a feeling
of superiority in doing this, over the one who received the money.

In the same manner the fanatic adherence to
truth in many neurotics proves itself to be, as a
rule, a reaction of the weaker against the superior power (in this connection the original picture of the same may be called, the *"enfant terrible"*).

I learned from the previous history of a catatonic that he was oppressed and humiliated by
his wife. One night he broke out in sobs and
told her that he had deceived her by an affair
with a servant girl. His masculine protest made
use of this expedient, adultery, in order to connect with it an open confession. Again, in the

form of the neurotic conjunction with which we are already acquainted, it became apparent that the wife not only had the stronger will, but had, also, the command of the pocket-book. The patient, himself a weak man, was obliged to live from her revenues, something that the wife and her family made the source of much unpleasantness, though they knew all about it beforehand. In order to protect himself from the superiority of his wife and not to submit entirely to her influence, he, already engaged in conflict over the male domination, arrived at an arrangement of a psychic impotence. The wife, on the other hand, overcame this impotence and humiliated the husband openly. His flirtation with the nurse girl was the beginning of his revenge. This could only be effective in a way to elevate him if he confessed his adultery in a manly way; therefore he had recourse to the love of truth, which had already served him as a vehicle for all sorts of rascality. The fact that he confessed his fault with tears was in keeping with his cowardice before a decision, but on the other hand, made it easier for him to communicate the painful intelligence to his wife. The further course turned out against the masculine triumph of the psychic hermaphrodite; the wife went further in her aggression and complained to her relatives who in turn reproached him in the most severe manner.

Now he fell into an apathy with an augmented craving for security, wished to undo his transgression as it had not assisted him to the masculine triumph and found the solution in a fiction of a purifying miracle which God had wrought in him. He was again on the heights, his predestination phantasy broke out, he stood in communication with God, received orders and commands from Him, and built up a psychotic system in which he wandered on the earth as a prophet. The masturbation, too, which he practiced openly, he designated as a miracle, in order thus to escape the feeling of humiliation. Stereotypies were manifested, among other ways, by an occasional upright position of the body and by holding the head high, a motion which I was able to interpret as symbolic, as a phantasy of the erection of the male organ.

"To tell some one a bitter truth—" This expression contains the kernel for the comprehension of the case just described. The neurotic often makes use of the truth in order to cause pain to others. One never hears agreeable truths from neurotic patients without a reaction immediately becoming visible, usually in the form of an aggravation of the suffering. To every emotion of love, which is regarded as feminine, as a submission, there follows an emotion of hate, as masculine protest, the latter in the garments of truth—honor bright! Also in this case of dementia præcox we find a stage where the doubt of the neurotic concerning his own masculinity is bridged over by means of expedients and by a tightening of the guiding fiction where the compensatory craving for security gives the impulse to take a guiding symbol verbally and to construct the fiction (as if the neurotic were a teacher, the Emperor, Savior). Other traits, such as moodiness and unsociability, are likewise to be recognized as neurotic anticipatory preparations, as always fitted to annihilate the superiority of others and to prevent them from carrying out their will.

The neurotic individual is the typical kill-joy and peace destroyer. He is misled by his megalomaniac ideal in conditions of greatest uncertainty and is always busy trying to hypostasize and deify his own guiding line, and to cross those of others. These traits are also capable of a more extended application. The neurotic regards his inability to get along with others, his disturbing attacks, as proofs that others wish to injure him, and erects, as a protection, the wall of his principles within which his spirit of mastery is able to develop. Here emerge tendencies such as the desire to be alone, sometimes the desire to be buried; or pictures, such as being buried alive or concealed in the mother's body (Gruner).

At times I have discovered as a fulfillment of this wish to dominate in solitude, the habit of remaining a long time on the stool. Wholly in the same direction, i. e., of gaining the upper hand, the neurotic carries out his exaggerated yielding and adaptability, but the patient is in this always on the watch, although he tries, too, in this way to captivate those who are stronger, to deviate toward the more manly line and to enjoy his open triumph.

The inclination to daintiness furnishes the neurotic with the same readiness for conflict. By this means he can decry everything, secure himself against decisions and lay claim to his prerogative. He will be finicky in such instances as harmonize best with his tendencies and where he can gain the most advantages. In eating, in the choice of friends, in amorous relations, he secures to himself thereby a troublesome superiority. Every one is obliged to make allowances for him because he is sick, nervous. This trait of character rises to great performances as soon as the fear of the sexual partner, of marriage, makes use of it. No girl, no man, then amounts to anything, and a twisted ideal furnishes the neurotic with a point of support for the disparagement of every one. At other times and in other relations, this trait manifests itself as an arrangement, as the foresight of an individual who has not as yet conquered the weak point of his feeling of inferiority. He can also be moderate "when the wind blows from the northwest," when his will to power requires it. One of the universal methods of quieting children when they show discontent is by comforting them with a prospect of the future, when they will be big, grown up. One often hears children themselves say, "When I am grown up, I will . . ." The problem of growth engages the attention of children to an extraordinary extent and in the course of their development they are constantly reminded of it. It is thus in regard to the size of his body, the growth of his hair, of the teeth, and as soon as he comes to speculations concerning the sexual organs by the growth of the pubes and the genital organs. The entrance of the child upon his masculine rôle, of which we have often spoken, requires a distinct largeness of the person of the individual and of the parts of his body. Where this is denied him—and here we encounter again the basis of somatic inferiority, especially the causal rickets (thymus anomalies?), anomalies of the thyroid, of the sperm glands, hypophysis, etc.—the child has recourse on account of its desire for masculine value to the positing of the masculine protest. Then it acquires the heightened impulse to covetousness, envy, bragging, greed, activity, together with the acute feeling of contrast and begins to measure himself constantly with others, especially with the persons of importance in his environment, and finally with the heroes from tales and stories. Thus the individual comes to a wishful contemplation of the future and the phantasy incited by the craving for security fills all wishes.

CHAPTER IV

THE DEROGATORY TENDENCY TO DISPARAGE OTH-
ERS; OBSTINACY AND WILDNESS; THE SEXUAL
RELATIONS OF NEUROTICS AS A MEANS OF
COMPARISON; SYMBOLIC EMASCULATION;
FEELING OF BEING BELITTLED; EQUALITY TO
MAN AS A LIFE-PLAN; SIMULATION AND NEU-
ROSIS; SUBSTITUTE FOR MASCULINITY; IMPA-
TIENCE; DISCONTENT; INACCESSIBILITY

THE compulsive craving of the neurotic to fill
his egoistic ideal with the overvalued masculine
traits impels him, especially because of the obstacles of reality, to a change in the formula of
his guiding line, so that he attempts to attain the
goal which he values as equal to the masculine
goal by means of circuitous paths. What drives
him to a psychosis is his longing to realize an
unattainable ideal. Should he suffer a defeat
in the main line of his masculine protest, or
should he even anticipate such a defeat, he seeks
a substitute which he temporarily considers as of
equal value through an arrangement of intensified reassuring expedients. At this point there
begins as a rule that process of psychic transfor-

mation which we designate as neurosis, in so far
as the guiding fiction does not lead to a violation
of reality, the patient only feeling it as a disturbing element, as is the case in neurasthenia, hypochondriasis, anxiety and compulsion neuroses and
in hysteria.   In the psychosis the guiding masculine fiction appears disguised in pictures and
symbols of infantile origin.   The patient then
conducts himself no longer as if he wished to be
masculine, above, and as if he sought to attain
this end by every possible means, but through the
medium of anticipation as though he already had
attained all these ends and only indicates at first,
incidentally and in the manner of a foundation
(depression, persecutory and self-accusatory
ideas, ideas of poverty), that he is underneath,
unmanly, feminine.

For the sake of clarity, I will now proceed to
the description of some neurotic character traits
which tend in a direct line to the masculine egotistic ideal, or are so closely connected therewith
that they force themselves upon the understanding as only slight deviations of the masculine protest.   They have been generally regarded as active, masculine traits and the neurotic can thus
appeal to this general opinion in which there is
agreement.   But we have already endeavored to
show in previous chapters that in the construction
of masculine traits the choice of the fictitious goal

is dependent upon and guided only within circumscribed limits by the conscious understanding
of the neurotic or even of the critical observer.
He also makes use of such guiding lines which to
general logic do not always seem masculine, or at
least only in part so, such for example as coquetry, deception, etc. As the direct traits of
character in line with the masculine protest may
be emphasized, the frequently displayed tendency
to be a man through and through, courageous,
ready for attack, open, hard-hearted, cruel, to excel every one in strength, influence, power, wisdom, etc. When the fundamental feeling of inferiority demands stronger reassuring compensations—because of an expected defeat or the suspicion of one, this compensation ensues by a
strengthening of the readiness for conflict which
now strives toward the masculine feeling of superiority, often by circuitous and more abstract
ways, revealing simultaneous and often contradictory traits—after the manner of tricks and
artifices. It is then that the neurotic may manifest pliancy instead of obstinacy, or side by side
with it, or as the occasion may require it, traits of
exorbitant arrogance and modesty, roughness
and mildness, courage and cowardice, lust for
power and submissiveness, masculinity and femininity, all of which are used to gain security from
defeat or in order to permit him by circuitous

ways to enhance his own egoistic ideal or disparage that of others. That it is possible to conquer by weakness, submissiveness and modesty is shown in the example of women and by many examples in the history of the world.

The dominancy of the self-created deities, of the guiding fiction is always easily discernible and is revealed in the psychosis with unmistakable clarity. I will endeavor to show by means of a dream of a 22-year-old girl who was suffering from enuresis nocturna and in the daytime from frequent outbreaks of rage and ill-humor, who could get along with no one but me, and who often had suicidal ideas, that all of these phenomena, together with other traits of lust for power, of obstinacy or of anxiety were under the guidance of the masculine protest, and that this protest was dependent in turn upon a constitutional inferiority of the urinary organ, which in combination with ugliness and mental retardation gave the impulse to the compensatory exhibition of an exaggerated masculine guiding line. In order to make the case brief and comprehensible, I preface the remark that the patient had applied the realities of her childhood to a reassuring neurosis, had constructed the enuresis as an ever-ready expedient and always had recourse to this symptom when her egoistic feeling suffered a humiliation. In this case, too, there was manifested the colossal power of the tendency to disparagement in the arrangement of the seizures which drove the mother to a powerless despair, while at the same time the patient disparaged her mother in the usual form of an allusion by excusing herself from all fault and throwing the blame on another. The following dream shows this in a specially clear manner.

"My mother showed my friend the dirty cover of the bed. We began to quarrel. I say the cover is yours and begin to cry bitterly. I awake flooded in tears."

A short time before she related to me that she often awoke weeping from sleep without knowing the cause of her weeping. From the connection of the genesis of the disease which was apparent even at that time the weeping was of significance in relation to the mother, it represented one of the most usual childish procedures for diminishing the mother's superiority. After the communication of the dream she remarked, "You will certainly believe that you are right in your opinion concerning my weeping." One hears such remarks during a psychotherapeutic treatment as a regular thing, and must not overlook the concealed criticism therein as a device of the tendency to disparage, which is directed against everybody. The moderate expression of the same on this occasion led me to suspect that the cure of the neurosis was in progress, as the more lively reactions were absent. Formerly under similar circumstances she would have asserted sharply and passionately that I was wrong, or she would have omitted to mention or would have forgotten those dreams which confirmed my view. I was further confirmed in my assumption by the information that the patient after the dream immediately took off the slightly soiled bed linen and washed it in secret which was never the case before because the sight of the soiled linen was intended for her mother.

For the explanation of the dream she related the following. She was firmly convinced that her mother told all her acquaintances about her enuresis. All her relatives seemed to know of her weakness. Once an uncle, obviously in order to comfort her, had informed her that both he and another brother had for a long time been in the habit of wetting the bed. In her dreams she reproached her mother, telling her, *"The weakness is in your family, you are to blame if I soil the bed, the soiled cover is yours."*

She related further that in changing she often took a bed-slip instead of a cover; the one was closed, the other open; adding, "And it is easy to mistake them in the closet."

Behind this thought lies the problem of open

and shut which is clearly recognizable as an expression for the oppositeness of the sexes. She blames her mother for the disease, but at the same time casts, so to speak, a furtive glance at its source and spring, that is, the femininity for which she blames her mother and betrays to us in the masculine protest of her dreams how slightly she estimates the difference between man and woman. Similarly George Sand declared that there was only one sex. The quarreling and weeping is the most important attitude of her aggression against her mother whose superiority she tried to destroy in this way as well as by her adherence to the enuresis. The fact that at the present time she operates against men by her enuritic device and thereby avoids marriage and "the tyranny of man," is a natural result to be inferred from other perspectives of her neurotic psyche.

An example of the change of formula of the guilding masculine fiction which originally was "I will be a man," in the above described stage of the treatment was, "I will be superior to my mother like a man," and later on was expressed in the words, "I will humiliate my mother by feminine means." In a dream, therefore, in a tentative, anticipatory test, this guiding line as we have maintained it to be comes to stronger expression. The dream is as follows:

*"I lie in a burning bed.   All weep about me.
I laugh aloud."*

A discussion of free love had preceded the
dream.   The burning bed, according to the patient's interpretation represented amorous pleasure.   We translate according to our understanding of the dream.   "How would it be if I should
embrace free love?   Then my mother would be
humiliated but I would laugh at her, would be
superior to her."   Attention must also be called
to the expression "burning," which arises so frequently in psychic constructions which spring
from the urinary functions in antithesis to water
(enuresis). [1]

The laughing in this dream is equivalent to the
weeping in the first dream.   Both show the aggressive tendency which seeks the mother's defeat.   In this case, too, the untenability of the
assumption of a splitting of personality is readily
perceivable.   Just as erroneous would be the assumption of a real sexual wish.   This means
would only serve the purpose of the patient if the
mother were set back and she could play the part
of man in regard to her.

The guiding fiction of the equality to man
comes to expression in some way or other in all

[1] Adler, "Studie," l. c., Addendum.   Freud has already touched
upon the relationship between fire and water in the dream, and the
allegorical representation based on this.

women and girls. As I was able to show in the foregoing case, it is the change of formula necessitated by reality which disguises the masculine protest. Hence it is essential in the analysis of neurotic female patients to discover at what point they protest against their femininity. This point can always be found, for the pressure toward the maximation of the ego-consciousness necessitates the construction of a reassuring guiding line which is erected as an antithesis to the idea "feminine." Cultural or uncultural ideas of emancipation, of militancy directed against men and their privileges are usually found in normal women and girls. They seek to diminish the distance as much as possible in dress, attitude, customs, laws, views of life. The masculine protest of neurotics is exaggerated in all these directions. In dress glaring but at the same time mannish fashions are affected, as the lengthening of single parts of dress and the wearing of strong high shoes. Or they avoid all fashions in dress which are distinctly feminine. Often there is a lively fight against the corset, a fight directed against the confinement, but which can also serve other purposes and is often brought into play to avoid seeing company and is most usually directed against the husband. The attitude and habits of neurotic women are often so masculine that it is noticeable from the first moment. Crossed legs

and arms, and at times only indications which
betray this tendency, as well as the tendency to
take the left side as a man does or to allow no one
to stand in front of them, etc., as in the dream.
In the neurotic's view of life the usual ideal overestimation of the masculine qualities is compensated for in a practical manner by the disparagement of men. In sexual relations anasthesia is
the rule. Masculine variants, or those which disparage man are given preference.

The neurotic psyche of men offers the same
characteristics. It derives its artifices from an
imaginary consciousness of femininity in order to
arrive at a feeling of complete manliness. One
of my patients who was suffering from asthma
nervosum presented a very clear example of this
dynamic. He had been a weak child and had
suffered from the exudative diathesis, a relation
to which Strümpell has called attention. His
early catarrh permitted him already in childhood
to press his mother into his service. She took him
to her, cared for him in her bedroom and yielded
to all his wishes. He was early placed under the
care of a strict governess of whom he could not
get the better, notwithstanding his rage and in-
tractibility. He felt weak before her and thus
became acquainted with childish deceptions by
means of which he was able to escape the governess, that is, he simulated and exaggerated the

catarrhal affection by an arrangement of coughing and excitation of the bronchial tubes and
larynx and by asthmatic phenomena which he
produced after the manner of straining at difficult defecation, by tension of the abdomen and
closing of the anus. He soon learned to know
that these phenomena gained him a place in his
mother's room, and in the course of years produced an asthmatic device which he was to set unconsciously into activity whenever he felt compelled on account of his overtense fictitious guiding goal to rise to the position of the lord of the
house, and incidentally, of the governess. He
soon gained the victory so that the governess was
forbidden to treat him severely or to beat him.

We see how his egotistic ideal had at its disposal from now on a neurotic weapon which
placed him in a position to escape a defeat or to
prevent the emergence of the feeling of his
original inferiority in a circuitous way, that is, no
longer by obstinacy, rage, courage, manliness, but
that he sought to get ahead by a sort of treachery,
craft, unmanly conduct, cowardice, a leaning on
the mother. This subterfuge, hypostasized and
elaborated to an unconsciously working mechanism, furnished him the necessary security for his
whole life. His neurotic symptom which was
constantly defended and laid claim to by further
auxiliary lines of his trait of character, i. e. "to

possess everything" by his lust for power, by his
obstinacy and disputatiousness, and at the same
time by his cowardice, fear of new undertakings,
fear of men and women and by the tendency to
disparagement which always evolves from these
traits and which played such an important rôle in
his aggressive devices furnished him a new organ,
a means of making himself important in a special
way, to dominate his world, inasmuch as he could
always demand the protection of his mother. He
felt safer with his mother than with his wife, and
thus he was driven by necessity to fall in love with
his mother, a love which upon closer analysis
proved to be a sort of tyranny. Pregnancy
phantasies reflected for him the feelings of humiliation connected with a feminine rôle and alter-
nated with thoughts about castration and with
phantasies about being a woman. His impulse
to masturbation revealed the attempt to emanci-
pate himself victoriously from women, to avoid a
defeat, to conduct himself in a manly fashion, and
was continued in similarly directed phantasies of
greatness, both of which were forms of expression
of his masculine protest. The imagined smallness of his genital organs, a thought which made
a marked impression upon him, served him as a
figure and perceptional form for his inferiority
and feminine nature. From his childhood he
sought to attribute all his unsuccessful efforts and

defeats to his small penis, apperceived and grouped his experiences in this direction and according to related antithetical forms of apperception of "manly-womanly." The small penis represented to him the figurative marginal concept between masculinity and femininity and was manifestly constructed as was the attitude of the patient on the idea of a corporal and psychic hermaphroditism and its tragedy. It is no wonder that in the psycho-analysis of these cases with the male-female manner of apperception which belongs to the foundation of the neurotic psyche, one hits only upon sexual relations. They are all to be understood as a *modus dicendi,* as a jargon, and figurative modes of expression and are to be resolved into forms, whereby strength, victory, triumph come to expression in male sexual symbols, defeat in female and the neurotic artifices in both together, usually also in a perverse or hermaphroditic symbolism.

It was easy to detect in our patient that besides the sexual mode of expression he had another fashion of apperception based upon the antithetical formula of inspiration-expiration which had been set in operation by the inferiority of his respiratory organ inclusive of the nose. Even the speech used for our mutual understanding likewise made use of such formulæ and a sigh of relief from an oppressed breast could very well

be clothed in the figure of "having air again."
The patient was also able to represent, in pantomime form, memories of his boyhood race, a wild
race to get to first place, the desire to be the first
at the goal by means of breathless efforts.   In a
dream during the latter part of the treatment he
made use of his ability to whistle (which is to be
understood figuratively) in order to accentuate
his manliness by respiration.   The dream was as
follows:

*"It seemed to me that four people were whist-
ling. I remark that I can do it just as well as
they."*

A short time before he had begun a relation
with the governess in the family of his married
brother and had asked her the question if his
brother often visited his wife at night.   The girl
answered in the negative.   Being able to whistle
is the ideal of all small boys and some girls make
efforts to acquire this manly attitude.   In his
dream he made a tentative comparison to see if he
was the equal of his male relatives and thus arrived from this line, which originated in his feeling of effeminacy, to the masculine protest.   He
is the equal of all four.

In this case too I found my observation confirmed that the neurotic feels his sexual libido,
and manifests the same only in accordance with

the manner and degree that is required by his
fictive goal, so that every psychological opinion
which perceives in the libido a constitutionally acquired factor, in its alterations and fortunes the
essence of the neurosis, becomes untenable. It is
especially easy to arrange sexual and excitations
and they are always in some way subordinated
to the masculine protest. The identification of
masculinity with sexuality takes place in the neurosis by means of abstraction, symbolization and
a figurative somatic-jargon, and it is this false
artifice of the neurotic which fills his thought content with sexual pictures.

The contentiousness and hidden querulousness
which stand in the closest relation to the tendency
to disparagement present difficult tactical and
pedagogic problems to the psychotherapeutist.
They betray in every case the weak point, the
feeling of inferiority of the patient which drives
him to compensation. It is easy to uncover this
neurotic aggressiveness by a very simple mode of
approach. Let it be imagined that the neurotic
feels that he has entirely lost his masculinity and
feels himself humiliated and now let it be noted
through what artifice he seeks to carry out the
completion of his character or his overcompensation. One will then find a number of preparatory devices, characteristics, syndromes and sym-
toms which have for their aim the representation

of an ideal organ, but one must however be prepared to view this as a riddle, which requires solution. For this "ideal organ," namely—the neurosis or psychosis, is of masculine origin and has for its purpose the prevention of a lowering of the patient's ego-consciousness, and to bring him closer to his masculine goal. Cruel reality, however, impedes the development of this fiction to such an extent that the most peculiar circuitous ways must be resorted to so that partial and apparent results are striven after without bringing the patient nearer to his goal. Without the help of the psychotherapeutist who in rare cases may prove to be a substitute for the fortunes of life, this "will to seem" becomes more and more accentuated in case of failure, and constantly strengthens the abstract, main line of the old guiding fiction. One of the principal circuitous ways along which this ideal organ—i. e. the masculine protest,—works, is the tendency to disparagement. That is the reason that it has been mentioned so often because it attracts the attention of the physician and is an expression of the strength of the neurotic impulse. It likewise furnishes an ever-present point of contact by means of which it may be possible to instil some insight into the patient and it is at the bottom of those phenomena which Freud has described as resistance and has falsely viewed as the result of repressed sexual excitations. With this tendency the neurotic comes to the physician and he carries it with him, as does also the normal person, when he returns home. Only that then his increased insight stands as a guard, warning him against giving expression to this tendency and thus the patient is forced to show his desire to be "first" in other ways.

One should never hesitate to guard all expressions of doubt, of critique, of forgetfulness, of tardiness, all demands of the patient, relapses after improvements, continued silence, as well as adherence to symptoms as effective means of the tendency toward disparagement directed against the psychotherapeutist. One will rarely err in proceeding thus and usually be justified in this opinion by the comparison of coincident phenomena of a similar trend. The expressions of these tendencies are often of the most subtile nature. Shall I add that the most extensive experience and knowledge in regard to this "tendency to disparage" is barely sufficient to prevent being taken by surprise, and that a great deal of tact, renouncement of authority, and even friendliness, watchful interest and the consciousness of being in the presence of a sick person with whom it is out of place to engage in strife are indispensable to good results?

I found it necessary once to explain to a stuttering patient the position of the larynx, by means of a drawing. Instead of taking the drawing home with him as he had intended in order to give it further consideration, he left it with me on the table. The next day he was a quarter of an hour late, first went to the toilet, related something of another patient who had complained of me, and after some silence related a dream which ran as follows:

"It seemed to me that I had been looking at a drawing. A cylinder extended out from a circle; it did not run straight but sideways."

The interpretation showed that this dream had reference to the drawing of the larynx on which the larynx was drawn straight downwards. The patient argued with me in the dream as though he would say "How would it be if my physician were wrong?" and thus revealed to me his distrustful attitude—the fear of being deceived and at the same time the tendency to disparagement directed against me, which had been revealed by the subconscious measures of the forgetfulness, the delay, the recital of the complaint, the silence, and finally by the tentative endeavor in the dream to put me in the wrong. One may justly expect that the patient applies his stuttering for the same purpose against me and will continue thus to use it. In spite of many contradictions he forced me into the rôle of a former teacher whom he often corrected, so that he could continue to use against me his former artifices.[2] This was revealed by his remarks concerning his dreams and further from the fact that his disease was assumed and adhered to in order to decry his father and gain superiority over him.

A female patient who was assigned to me for treatment because of depression, suicidal ideas, weeping fits and "lesbischen Neigungen" was sent by me after a brief course of treatment because of the suspicion of a genital affection, to a gynecologist who removed a large myoma and prognosticated a cure of the neurosis from the operation. After the operation the patient journeyed to her home and from there wrote me that the gynecologist was right in his prognosis. Of course she added it was to be expected that the operation succeeded better in the case of a countess upon whom the same surgeon had operated, and of whom she had read in the papers, than it had in her case. Soon afterward she visited me, argued against one of my contributions which she had in some way procured, declared her extreme interest in my method of treatment, said her condition was the same as before the operation and vanished. From the portion of her his-

[2] An artifice which had for its purpose a tendencious, derogatory, affective expression.

tory which she communicated to me during the treatment it became apparent among other things that she lived at swords-points with her whole environment, that she dominated her husband entirely, that she hated the village and played the man psychically and sexually to one of her friends. Her fear of the blessing of children was astounding, sexual relations unbearable because her husband seemed too heavy. When the latter visited her once during the treatment, she had the day before his visit the following dream:

"It seemed to me that the whole room was enveloped by fire."

She gave the information spontaneously that this was a typical dream, and that it always returned at the time of her menstrual period. This time it occurred a long time before her period. The dream could be easily recognized as an attempt to use a feminine situation, menstruation, for the purpose of the masculine protest— that is to avoid sexual relations. A deeper penetration into the meaning which would certainly have revealed an enuresis in childhood (fire-myoma see "Studie," Appendix) was prevented by the interruption of the treatment. I received another letter which contained the assurance that the patient from now on would try to find peace in her environment in my sense of the word. I think that this must have been still difficult for her.

Obstinacy, wildness and unruliness may in the same way serve as the proof which female patients seek in order to show how little they are fitted for the feminine rôle. These preparations begin already in the earliest childhood and lead gradually to physical and psychic aptitudes in gestures, facial expression, emotional predispositions and mimicry, while the character develops in the direction of the ideal guiding line and cautiously introduces the patients' attitude of life. In many cases these characteristics are manifested in a direct manner and serve without deviation for the expression of the masculine protest. Or there takes place a change of formula in the guiding fiction, either because of the emergence of contradictions in the guiding line, in the event of a real or threatened defeat, or because of something that usually coincides therewith, namely, an obstacle of reality which is estimated as unsurmountable. Under the construction of a security-giving anxiety or feeling of guilt, or security-giving antithetical traits (dissociation of other writers), the deviations in neurotic circuitous ways follow. But the preparatory devices persist. It is only that the neurotic cautiousness introduces the devia—under these new forms of security, anxiety, feeling of guilt, seizures, when the patient would otherwise have had to answer with the originally developed emotions such as, anger, rage, aggression. Frequently there come to light purposefully grouped memory pictures of a certain "boundlessness," thoughts, memories, illusions as though one were boundlessly desirous, sensuous, demoniac, criminal, are manifested, at times obviously arranged oversights and accidents which are nothing else than admonitions to be cautious. Or the sudden termination of the direct masculine aggressiveness takes place always just before a decision, a peculiarity which characterizes many neurotic love affairs. The deviation in such cases from the direct guiding line may follow in a perverse manner under the influence of the craving for security, or the guiding line leads him to seek the protection of the father, mother, God, alcoholism or an idea. Attempts to reach the top through feminine means, or to surpass at least, all women, leads to excessive cleanliness, to the "cleaning mania," to a masochistic subjection or coquetry, to a desire to please and in female patients to a constant fretting. Along with this there will always be found character-traits and tell-tale traces which betray that the masculine fiction is all-powerful and seeks to arrive at its purpose by these circuitous ways. The excessive eroticism in many of these cases is not to be understood as real, that is to say, as depending upon a constitutional basis but shows itself to be associated with the fiction, and to be due to an uninterrupted attentiveness which has taken an erotic direction. The same is true of perversions and an apparently weakened libido, which are constructed from neurotic subterfuges. All sexual relations in the neurosis are only a simile.

The fear of the superiority of the male and the depreciatory struggle directed against it is often clothed, as result of the neurotic antithetical perspective, in phantasies of emasculation which have for their object the deprivation of the male of worth. In the dreams of these female neurotic patients this comes clearly to light and can be readily proved by coexistent derogatory tendencies. One of these dreams is here given. The patient came under my care shortly after she had undergone an operation for a fistula, because of a compulsory thought and excitement. The compulsory thought ran, "I will never be able to attain anything." At our very first meeting she expressed the thought whether I would be able to attain anything. The same line of disparagement illuminated her dream. She dreamed, *"I cried out in my dream, Marie, the fistula is there again."* The surgeon had promised her complete recovery and kept his word. He is under obligations to her in many ways and did not wish to take a fee. The patient became very excited over this and regarded it as an humiliation. For some time after she tortured herself with plans for paying the debt. Her servant was called Marie, and she had never spoken to her about the operation. If there should take place a new breaking out of the fistula her first trip would be to the surgeon to whom she would express her opinion. Marie, a female servant becomes the surgeon. The patient imagines the circumstances demanded by her masculine egoistic feeling, the surgeon has operated poorly, has not kept his promise, is a woman and a servant at the same time. This expresses the way in which she could attain everything if she were only a man.

When one examines the published analyses of no matter what psychological school the mechanism of the neurotic masculine protest will always be found therein. I shall again emphasize this in connection with the analysis of a case of migraine.

The patient related immediately from the reminiscences of her childhood that she had constantly lived in conflict with her elder brothers because they wished to dominate her. This sort of reminiscences led, as soon as they were voluntarily related, to a hidden contest against male domination, and one will never be deceived in the assumption that other character-traits also point to this strife to become equal to the male. Uninfluenced, our patient continued to relate that she played almost exclusively with boys and was treated by them as one of their kind. This method of expression betrayed very clearly the high estimation in which the male sex was held, which brought this girl nearer to her father— something which may easily be interpreted as sexual love for the father and as the "incest complex."

The development of our patient took the same course. She took her father wholly as her ideal; especially as she once caught her mother in a lie she was anxious to imitate her father's example of truthfulness and punctuality.[3] She remembered also that her father had often regretted that she was not a boy, and that it was his wish that she should study. In this situation an egoistic feeling was naturally developed in which ambitious efforts could not be absent. On the other hand her bashfulness which wrecked many of her principles was very noticeable to herself and others. This bashfulness is found with extraordinary frequency in the histories of neurotics. It is identical with the feeling of uncertainty, as soon as this is manifested in relations with others. Blushing, stuttering, downcast looks, avoidance of the society of adults, excitement before examinations

[3] What other authors term imitativeness, identification, is always to be looked upon as the assumption of a *model* for the purpose of a heightening of the ego-consciousness.

and stage fright often accompany the attempts at approaches to other people or at the establishment of relations with them.   Analysis shows that the feeling of inferiority is the source of this sort of uncertainty, usually accompanied by a strong feeling of shame.   The feeling of inferiority is conditioned by somatic inferiority which makes itself felt psychically, by faults of childhood and strong psychic pressure on the part of parents and relatives, and finally by real or imagined femininity which develops early in strong contrast to a male member of the family (father or brother).   The analogy according to which the most diverse emotions of being belittled, of humiliation, of inferiority are apperceived by the child is then usually the analogy of "the smallness of the penis," which is to be understood symbolically, and thoughts of castration develop, of a feminine rôle in sexual relations, of conception and pregnancy or of persecution, of being stabbed or wounded, of falling and being "beneath."   All these fictions are revealed in day-dreams, hallucinations, dreams, in so far as they are not wholly supplanted by the fiction of the masculine protest and express a feeling of being belittled, which breaks forth in the thought, "I am a woman," against which the egoistic feeling presses forward and the masculine protest struggles.

Of our patient we hear that she had some

knowledge of sexual relations at a time when from lack of experience she was unable to take into account its results and purposes. In such cases we may always expect to find bashfulness, shame and doubt, and in later years fear of tests and decisions in every form, traits of character which resolve themselves analytically into the idea that others might be able to discover on the person of the patient genital defects or omissions. The characteristics which display an effort to attain equality with the male sex are usually manifested at an early age, and this effort occupies the foreground, while in many cases because of a tinge of hopelessness "the innate coloring of the decision" is affected. Because the direct route to masculinity is closed or seems to be so, circuitous and deviating ways are sought out. On one of these circuitous ways lies the socially valuable effort of woman toward emancipation, on another, the private expression of the masculine protest, the neurosis of woman, the construction of the ideal male organ.

It was easy to see in the case of this patient that in her childhood she had sought to attain the domination of man, of her brothers and her father, as she apparently had made very short work of her mother. Her father fell entirely under her authority. After a little experience the conclusion is easily arrived at concerning the

direction of her neurotic symptoms, that her
headache and migraine represent since her marriage a means for gaining the mastery over her
husband. And in this mastery she sought a substitute for her masculine power which she believed to have lost.

I know the objection which might be raised at
this point. How shall the severe suffering of a
neurosis, the terrible pain of trigeminal neuralgia, insomnia, unconsciousness, paralysis, migraine all be thrown into the bargain merely as a
means to an end, because of the failure to attain
equality with man? I have myself struggled
against this conviction which thrust itself upon
me. Is the case very much different when human
beings endure all sorts of hardships for a whole
life time in order to attain some other worthless
bubble? Furthermore, as I have already shown,
on these neurotic circuitous paths to masculinity
are found also crime, prostitution, the psychosis,
suicide. This in addition to the mystery which
shrouds human psychic mechanisms may be cited
in support of my understanding of the matter.
The psychic therapy of the neuroses is certainly
based upon an understanding of the exaggerated
valuation of the male destiny. And I draw from
this objection the advantage in regard to my patients inasmuch as I endeavor to show them how
they, placed before a choice between a natural

rôle and the neurotic masculine goal, choose the greater of the two evils.

From the previous history of our patient the further facts may be emphasized that she always had a disinclination to play with dolls, furthermore that until her marriage she took the greatest pleasure in gymnastics and sports. That these efforts too, served as a substitute for masculinity is manifested more from their connection with other masculine traits than from their own nature, more especially from a sort of importunity with which the patient spoke of them. She was also passionately fond of extensive touring, of which inclination since the birth of her child, whom she wished and expected to be male, only the desire to make occasional journeys remained.

The error must be avoided, however, of assuming that the traits of character here described and emphasized by the patient herself formed isolated islands in the extensive soul-life of a woman. On the contrary, it must be assumed that these masculine traits came to expression under the pressure of a dominating tendency, had their origin in a distinct life-plan and became conspicuous phenomena only because they had the power to do so, while all around these phenomena there existed an indistinct, only occasionally manifested masculine craving which was principally occupied with the prevention and transformation of feminine emotions until such time as it shall have reached an independent existence. In this conflict of masculine against feminine emotions the egoistic feeling is thrown entirely on the side of masculinity and makes use even of persistently emerging feminine emotions, among others also of the female sexual appetite in order to collect them as humiliating and dangerous,[4] to group them, to exaggerate, to emphasize them and at the same time to surround them with sentinels so that they may be robbed of their influence. These sentinels, securities, usually extend beyond the sphere of feminine emotions. One always finds that these reassurances and protective devices, among which should be placed our symptoms of disease, do not stop at the mere fulfillment of their destiny, that is, the avoidance of defeat, but that they permeate these patients with a sort of cautiousness which finally renders them unfit for anything. It is only then that the primary insecurity which may be likened to a fear of a feminine rôle is at an end, but by this time it has permeated the entire life-relation of the individual and forces him outside the realm of all social relationship. We find all our patients in the midst of this retreat and their

[4] This affective accentuation is always derived from a purposeful device. Feminine rôle and abyss, drowning, death, being run over, or strangled.

symptoms are for them assurances that they will not be forced back into the tumult of life. From this there develops a neurotic picture which often reveals a reversion to simpler, more child-like relations, either because these are developed after maturity, or for the reason that maturity was generally impeded. Thus many act as though they were in the nursery. Family relations become accentuated to an extraordinary degree, or instead of childish love for the parents the old childish obstinacy develops and both factors are used as guiding symbols, as though the patient sought to discover in all persons the father or mother. Notwithstanding the fact that he comes in conflict with reality on account of this fiction, the patient holds fast to it because he found security in the relations existing in the nursery. Kipling relates of a person lying in the death struggle, whom he observed until the expected cry for the mother came from his lips. One has only to listen to the street-Arabs, who, when hard pressed, immediately cry out for their mother, in order to comprehend this longing for security. The same longing for security has crept into the worshipping of the Mother of God. In girls, the longing for security is as a rule in more pronounced analogy to the relation to the father. The "uterine phantasy" which is placed in the foreground by G. Grüner I have also found employed by neurotics only when they wish to express that peace can be found only with the mother, or when they have thoughts of suicide, that is, the wish to return to the same state in which they were before birth. (The hermaphroditic progression backward.)

Our patient, too, as child and girl sought this leaning on her father who spoiled her not a little. The mother, as is often the case, was more attracted to her brothers. This trait also shows itself to be conditioned by the exaggerated estimation of the masculine principle, which the father, being a man, would more readily renounce in her favor. Our patient soon noticed that her father's care for her increased whenever she was ill. Thus she came to have a special preference for being sick, which procured for her further petting, love, and sweetmeats. She must have regarded as the most appropriate substitute for that manliness which she believed to be lost to her, that condition of sickness which gained for her the command of the whole house, the gratification of all her wishes and permitted her to escape all unpleasant encounters in school and society. Yes, it meant for her the highest attainable potency, her feeling of security, as soon as her father believed that she was ill. And she sometimes pretended to be ill, that is, she simulated or exaggerated.

best insight into this condition not from a neurotic symptom, but from a borderline case. We mean the psychology of sympathy. We are in a position to feel the suffering of another person as if it affected our own corporal sphere. Yes, we can even feel the suffering of another in anticipation before its occurrence. Well known examples of this are the anxious feelings which many persons experience when they see others, servant girls, roof workers or circus actors in dangerous situations, or even when they only think of such situations. These symptoms are usually felt by those who suffer from dizziness when in high places and they act when others are in danger exactly as though they themselves stood at a window or on a rock. They withdraw under the feeling of anxiety, placing a safe distance between themselves and the usually not dangerous position, in short, they have a feeling akin to that which they would have were they themselves in a dangerous position. Here the exaggerated cautiousness becomes apparent which in neurotics is so strong that they will not cross a bridge for fear that they might fall into the water or throw themselves into it. I have found similar mechanisms of cautiousness in all cases of fear of places and they reveal to us that we have a patient who wishes to avoid decisions, who fears whether he is equal to a certain situation, usually the sexual partner. In all other phobias, too, as I have shown in my description of syphilidophobia, (Zeitschr. f. Psych., Bd. I, Heft 9, 1911), this "sympathy" in a situation which has not as yet been realized, but which may be expected with probability constitutes the characteristic symptom (Lipps). It reveals itself as a very efficient tool of the craving for security, takes the place in many cases of a morality which is not invincible in character. Careful examination of this character-trait reveals that it has its foundation in that sort of feeling-participation for purposes of security, which is clearly set forth in Kant's categorical imperatives for the expression of the whole character, when this philosopher wishes each single individual to be influenced in his action by a point of view which permits of being regarded *as if* it were elevated to a universal maxim.[6]

Fictions, maxims, guiding principles then similar to the reassuring fictions of the simulator form part of the mental character of all persons, especially of neurotically inclined children. And reduced to their nucleus all of these formulæ are as follows: Act as though you were a complete man, or wished to be one. The content of this procedure which usually turns out to be in the nature of a substitute is determined beforehand by the experience of the child and by the special

6 Vaihinger, "The Philosophy of As If."

type of somatic inferiority from which he suffers, but is subject to special alterations which must be regarded as formal changes arising from special circumstances connected with experiences to which he gives neurotic valuations.

Somatic inferiority determines through the accompanying psychic phenomena of repugnance the direction of the ideas of pleasure and thus conducts the compensatory processes into the psychic regions. Here, too, we behold the craving for security at work and usually in such a purposeful manner that it works coefficients which offer security and thus gives rise to an over-compensation.[7] In the development, for instance of the stuttering Demosthenes to the greatest orator of Greece, of Clara Schumann, who was deaf to an accomplished musician, of the near-sighted G. Freitag, of many poets and painters with anomalies of the eye to visually talented persons and of the numerous physicians with anomalies of hearing, we perceive the result of the craving for security. We likewise see the result in every weak child who wishes to be a hero, in the clumsy child with thyroid affection who wishes to be an athletic racer and later in life always tries to be the first.

But the direction of the craving for security in order to have its objective point must depend

7 J. Reich, "Art and the Eye," Öst, Rundschau, 1909.

upon an example. And here the man offers more attraction to the egoistic feeling of childhood than does the woman. Indeed it seems that a female example can only be imitated after an initiatory conflict and only when this feminine example permits the attainment of mastery along the lines of least resistance.

This was the case with our patient as it often is with cases of migraine. Numerous writers have emphasized the circumstance that it is so often possible to trace the inheritance of migraine from the mother. We must give up the idea of the inheritance of migraine in the same manner as we were obliged to abandon the view of its organic etiology. I have already explained the nature of this question,[8] in the case of a seven-year-old girl and had before that been convinced that a feeling of uncertainty and humiliation precedes the attack of migraine, and that the attacks serve to place the whole household at the service of the sufferer, for which reason the example of the mother is imitated. The husband, the father, other relatives suffer no less from the attack than does the patient. Thus migraine is to be placed in the series of neurotic affections which serve to secure the mastery in the household and in the family. That this tyranny has a masculine significance and can be reduced to the wish to be a

[8] "Neurotische Disposition," Jahrbuch Bleuler-Freud, 1908.

man becomes obvious from further analysis. But a brief consideration of the migraine which occurs at the time of menstruation teaches us to understand in this case also the dissatisfaction with the feminine rôle. I have in various instances learned to recognize this connection with epilepsy, sciatica, trigeminal neuralgia. I have proved that these latter conditions in the cases mentioned by me were psychogenic in nature and originated whenever stronger securities were demanded.

The only sphere of influence which remained for our patient was her tyranny over her father, over whom she had complete power and this did not entirely satisfy her lust for power. Hence a "still, still more" declared itself as is often the case in neurotic affections and she sought a more obvious grasp of the subjugation of the father. Her mother suffered from migraine and the time of her attacks was, as is usual with patients suffering from migraine, a time of absolute power. Therefore our patient also who comprehended the value of the disease pretended to be suffering from it.[9] And our patient succeeded in doing what aboriginal man succeeded in doing when

9 In my work on "The Neurotic Disposition," I have already emphasized what must likewise be mentioned here, that an original somatic inferiority determines the choice of a symptom. In the neurosis the mechanism becomes the property of the psyche in the form of a disease-preparedness.

he made himself gods who filled him with terror, in creating for herself the migraine. This "as if" creation, this fiction became substantially independent, so that the pain and suffering could awaken whenever the patient needed them. The dramatic performance became so successful that the patient, because of its value in the direction of her tendencies, no longer saw through the fiction. Indeed she won by means of the same a superiority over and security against the husband just as she had previously done in regard to her father when she made use of this weapon to attain security. She strove to attain a masculine part in the marriage relation, directing all her activities towards gaining the mastery over her husband, but as there always remained an "and yet" it was necessary to obtain still further substitutes as evidences of power. And the most important of these substitute formations was the resolution not to have any more children. It had become a general principle in the household of this patient as in many others (one of which I described in the "Männliche Einstellung Weiblicher Neurotiker," Zeitsch., f. Psychoanalyse, Heft 4, 1910) that a woman who suffered from such headaches should have no more children. Insomnia, impossibility of going to sleep again after having been disturbed, references to the difficulties concerning the place of residence, various protective arrangements and the spoiling of the only child completed the security.

That these phenomena are merely a new view of the old wish for masculinity is proved by her first dream.

"I was at the depot with my mother. We wished to visit my father who was ill. I was afraid of missing the train. Then suddenly the father appeared. Then I was at a watch maker's and wanted to buy a substitute for the one I had lost."

She felt superior to her mother who was greatly respected by her, and also to her father who humored her slightest wish. Sick means weak. The father had died a short time previously. Shortly after his death she had one of her dreadful attacks of migraine. In the dream he came to life again and his person signified for her a maximating of her ego-consciousness. She had always been impatient, afraid of being late. Her brother came before she did and became a man. She felt spurred on to hasten (a man does it with one bound, a woman with a hundred), in order to arrive at the summit of her ego-consciousness. The day before the dream she was hastening to a concert and was held back by her mother. Women are often late and she did not wish to follow their example.

Reality reminded her nevertheless that she was a woman like her mother. The thought lies in the picture of being together with her mother at the depot. Her aggressive affect which is identical with the masculine protest is directed against her husband, against her father. In the further analysis of the dream the disparaging thoughts come to light, such as that the wife is stronger, more vigorous and healthier than the man. Then as a further incentive to conflict, the father (the man) suddenly emerges. This simile is taken from swimming and signifies in the neurotic perspective the "being above" in opposition to being "beneath." While the patient was afraid of missing the train, of being left behind in comparison with another, that is to say in comparison with the man, which can be supplied from the connection—to submit to him, she notices as her experience increases that the man is first, is above. The application of a picture, of an abstract idea in space for the purpose of illustrating the feeling of being belittled is often found in the neurosis, (See Syphilidophobia, l. c.) because it is adapted to prepare the disposition to conflict in the most extensive manner by means of the fictitious, abstract antithesis "nothing or all." In the same manner the artifice is made use of in painting, of representing the power of woman and the fear she inspires by giving her a higher position in space. In religious and cosmological phantasies this representation of superiority is the elevation of the position assigned. That in her dream the patient came through the spatially antithetical scheme according to the analogy of "man-woman," is indicated in the position of the patient beside her mother, that is, with her mother.

Thus the first dream which the patient had during the course of the treatment begins with considerations of masculine and feminine rôles. One should never neglect to take into consideration unprejudicially the possibility of the continuation of the dream and to await and compare new confirmatory data, even though the psychotherapeutist may have the most firm convictions concerning the significance of the problem for the neurosis. The further explanation of the patient was in regard to a watch chain which had been lost through the fault of her husband. She cannot remember having lost a watch. Interrogated concerning the significance in the dream of the watch which was substituted for the chain, the patient answered with considerable affect but evasively, that it was not the loss of the chain but of a charm attached to it that disturbed her. In short the watch hanging to a lady's chain is identical with the lost watch charm for which the patient grieves and for which she seeks a substitute.

The dream began with a symbolic contrast represented in space of an inferior femininity with a superior masculinity and ends with the logically following conclusion of the striving for a substitute for the lost masculinity. In this fictitious guiding line thus constructed the character, the affect reaction, the predispositions and neurotic symptoms must be represented, the correctness of which assumption the result of the case substantiated. The character-traits of impatience, discontent, obstinacy and reticence proved therefore to be, as did all the rest, auxiliary lines which stood in a dependent relation to the guiding fiction, that of attaining a masculine elevation.

CHAPTER V

CRUELTY. CONSCIENCE. PERVERSION AND NEUROSIS.

THE discovery of traits of a cruel nature in the very earliest childhood is unusually frequent in the course of an analysis of neuroses and psychoses. It would be wrong to apply our moral standards to the first two years of life, and to regard the activities of such children, who in reality are still incapable of either good or evil, as sadistic or brutal as it often happens when parents or guardians relate the histories of psychopaths. For these manifestations become psychic, or in our sense neurotic only when they begin to serve a definite end and are constructed as an abstraction which has some future tendency in view.[1] The fact that they are always created out of possibilities and capabilities of experience does not justify the assumption of a constitutional factor. As a matter of fact one only finds the character-trait of cruelty as a compensatory psychic construction in those children who, aside from this,

[1] See also Wagner v. Jaureg. "Ueber krankhafte Triebhandlungen," Wiener klin. Wochenschrift, 1912.

are forced by their feeling of inferiority to an early and hasty development of their *ideal of personality*. The accompanying traits of obstinacy, rage, sexual precocity, ambition, envy, greed, malice and delight in doing harm as they are regularly evoked by the guiding fiction, and which the strife and emotional predispositions help to form and mobilize, furnish the highly colored kaleidoscopic picture of the refractory child. The lust for power of such children is regularly manifested in the family life and play, but most of all in their bearing, attitude and glance. In the play and early thoughts concerning the choice of a vocation, the tendency to cruelty is often betrayed in a veiled manner and makes them regard as ideal types, the hangman, the butcher, the policeman, the grave digger, the savage or coachman, "because they can whip the horses," or the teacher, "because they can whip the children," the physician, "because they cut," or the soldier, "because they shoot," the judge, etc.[2]   The spirit of investigation is also often associated with this, and the torturing of animals and children, speculations and phantasies concerning possible misfortunes, often of those which might befall near relatives, an interest in funerals and church-yards and in horrible sadistic stories, are begun.

The first purpose of these exaggerated tenden-

[2] Adler, "Aggressionstrieb," l. c.

cies to cruelty, is to prevent the emergence and the becoming effective of the ever present possibility of weakness and pity, because these stand in opposition to the masculine guiding line. The general spreading of this craving to be manly which is thought to lead to superiority over others, is nowhere so clearly shown as in the disinterested pleasure in injuries. In neurotics this may be especially strongly emphasized and may be utilized in the most unreasonable manner for the purpose of exalting the ego-consciousness. La Rochefoucauld expresses this in his quaint manner as follows, "There is something in the misfortunes of our friends which is not quite displeasing."

I heard a patient laugh aloud when told of the Messina earthquake. He suffered from severe masochistic attacks. Compulsory laughter often possessed this patient when he was in the presence of a superior person, his teacher for instance, or some one who had some claim of authority over him. One finds in such patients a strong inclination to dominate over or torment others, at times sadistic phantasies, until one discovers that the compulsion to laughter, the lust for power and the sadism are erected over the weak point of the feeling of inferiority, in order to compensate for it. Pyromania, the delight in fire-brands and the almost irresistible compulsion to think of fire,

or to cry out "fire" in the theater or church seem
to be referable, according to certain of my findings, to defects of the sensitive bladder or to eyes
oversensitive to light, or at any rate to preparations for the compensation of these defects.   But
this guiding line of masculine cruelty is threatened with great danger and accident in a society
where there exist ethical imperatives, it can, therefore, be only followed in a disguised form.   Usually one sees deviations and circuitous paths in
following which the sadistic trait seems wholly or
in part lost.   In this way the neurotic succeeds in
gaining superiority over the weak, or he operates
on this new line so skillfully as to manage to set
up an aggression which enables him to dominate
and torture others.   In the compulsion neuroses
one frequently finds that these patients have
abandoned their sadistic guiding line and have
turned to penance and reassuring measures,
which have the same compulsory character and
are not less oppressive for the environment than
were the previous emotional predispositions of
the patient, and hence are fitted in the same manner as prime characteristics to render obvious the
superiority of the neurotic.   In the major attacks of so-called affective epilepsy, of hysteria,
of trigeminal neuralgia, of migraine, etc., the
masculine lust for power turns in the direction of
the neurotic "readiness for a paroxysm," but the

helplessness of the environment and its suffering is not less but rather greater than in the rages and enmity which were active ways of the neurotic. An inclination for antivivisectionism, vegetarianism, prevention of cruelty to animals, charity, often distinguishes these connoisseurs of the sufferings of others, they cannot endure to see a goose bleed, but clap their hands gleefully when their opponent leaves the Exchange a bankrupt. Their inclination to sectarianism forms an inimical antisocial trait, as does their severe criticism of the valuation of others which they exhibit before they even form an opinion of their own. Tolerance is unknown to them, unless they cry out for it for themselves.

If I sketch here traits which are to be encountered on all sides, they are nevertheless traits of a very prevalent neuroticism and signs of a deeply grounded uncertainty. They are by no means inherent in human nature, but are rather unsuccessful forms of the masculine protest which failed to bring assurance to the ego-consciousness. Should failure result in following the main guiding line, neurotic circuitous ways are entered upon and the "outbreak" of the neurosis or psychosis follows as a result of a change of form and accentuation of the guiding fiction.

I must also disagree with the theory of congenital criminality of children and criminals

promulgated by Lombroso and Ferrari, as well as
with Stekel's theory of the universal criminality
of neurotics. (Aggressionstrieb, l. c.). They
are nothing but forms of the aggressive impulse
become accentuated through the feeling of inferiority, and which makes use of the masculine guiding line. The transformation into a clearly obvious neurosis follows the abandonment of this
straightforward aggression. Where the fear of
a decision is absent, an early result of the security-giving neurosis, and where there develops a
strong tendency to deprive others of life, honor
and property, criminality is the result.[3]

In the developed neurosis, on the other hand,
one finds memory-traces of cruelty, criminality as
well as those of sexuality purposefully exaggerated, falsely grouped and retained. Through
the imagining of an accentuated conscience and
exaggerated feeling of guilt, the masculine protest is diverted from the straight path of aggression and becomes inclined towards routes of soft-
heartedness. It is only in the affect which occasionally comes to the surface, in the analysis of
the seizures, in the traits of character which become manifest now and then as is the case frequently at the onset of a psychosis and the nature
of the goal of the neurotic subterfuges and traits

[3] A. Jassny, "Dass Weib als Verbrecher," Arch. f. Kriminal-
psych., 1911, H. 19.

of character which have become diverted from the straight course, in the fact that a tyranny is erected in spite of all defeats, in the torture of others through self-torture, and finally in the intermixture of occasionally emerging original and direct traits of aggression, that one discovers the fact that the old over-tense goal still exists and that a change in the form of the fiction has only diverted the direction of the original tendency into other, often apparently opposite channels.

Thus it happens that following a decidedly aggressive period, the greedy, brutal or violent traits of the psychopath, in anticipation of a defeat or after such has actually been experienced, may be made to approach more closely or even too eagerly general moral ideals, through the construction of a fictitious factor, "conscience," in the same manner as the path of egocentric evil desire was entered upon from a feeling of inferiority. "Then I am destined to be bad," in this and similar ways the fictitious life-plan of many neurotics is unconsciously formed, until a glance into the abyss tears the giddy subject from his perilous position and forces him to seek a stronger security than is actually needed.   Conscience develops out of the simpler forms of prevision and self-evaluation under the pressure of the craving for security, is endowed with the attributes of power and raised to a divinity, so that the individual may construct his ideal without objection from any side, so that he may be able better to orient himself in the uncertainty of events and have his choice in attacks and methods of combat to which his will to power guides him.

But the neurotic brings about a reconstruction of his traits of character even for the sole purpose of being enabled to initiate the struggle to better advantage. Such is the case when he ascribes to the sexual partner of whom he stands in fear, traits of an egotistic, cruel and deceptive nature. He is then likely to hunt out and exaggerate from his memories and emotions, those which confirm his own character as affectionate, mild and open. For the purpose of proving these characteristics he will often act as though his virtues had the reality of innate and indestructible qualities.

One important question must still be touched upon. Nearly all of our neurotic patients come to us in the "stadium of virtue," after having experienced a defeat, and we must therefore expect to discover their masculine protest less in direct traits of character and emotional predispositions than in neurotic circuitous ways, accentuated security devices, which may be detected only with difficulty through the analysis of their dreams and symptoms. One will discover that the infantile, fictive guiding line has only become more effective, and in so far as it concerns the cases just spoken of, that their neurotic symptoms lead to a more intense degradation of others than did their original cruelty and desire to torture. For all these guiding lines are tensely stretched between the insecurity of the constitutionally or subjectively defective individual and his unattainable ego-ideal. However far back into childhood sadism, perversions of various sorts, sexual-libido, in short the masculine protest may extend, they are always constructed according to a life-plan and reveal their dependence thereon. The liberation of the sadism from the neurotic predisposition, and in the sense of Freud, from the unconscious and from repression, is to be likened to a carrying back of the neurosis to an earlier stadium, to a time before the defeat. Freud's scientific work, important and full of results as it was for the understanding of the neurosis, did not give a correct picture of the neurotic psyche. The neurotic predispositions of heightened affectivity, the exaggerated aggressiveness, the hypersensibility, and the direct, compensatory character-peculiarities require a liberation from their over-tense state; as do also the inclinations to neurotic perversions which are often constructed at a very early age, and which are to come to the aid of the general fear of decisions through a compromise formation. For this reason the effort should be made to conquer this feeling of inferiority and the tendency to disparage which results therefrom, these two important poles of every neurotic state, by means of insight and contemplation on the part of the patient, for they like their sexual analogies, (sadism, masochism, fetichism, homosexuality, incest-phantasies, apparent heightening or weakening of the sexual impulse), already form the foundation of the neurosis.

CHAPTER VI

THE ANTITHESIS ABOVE-BENEATH, CHOICE OF A
PROFESSION, SOMNAMBULISM, ANTITHESIS IN
THOUGHT, ELEVATION OF THE PERSONALITY
THROUGH THE DISPARAGEMENT OF OTHERS,
JEALOUSY, NEUROTIC AUXILIARIES, AUTHOR-
ITATIVENESS, THINKING IN ANTITHESES AND
THE MASCULINE PROTEST, DILATORY ATTI-
TUDE AND MARRIAGE, THE TENDENCY UP-
WARD AS A SYMBOL OF LIFE, COMPULSION TO
MASTURBATION, THE NEUROTIC STRIVING FOR
KNOWLEDGE

THE abstraction of the concept, "above-beneath," obviously plays an extremely important
rôle in the civilization of mankind, and is probably even connected with the beginning of the upright carriage of human beings. As every child
repeats this process in the course of his development when he arises from the floor and as training
also teaches him a disgust for clinging to the floor
and creeping on it from hygienic reasons, for being "down"; this higher development in childhood
may contribute not a little to the tendency to
value "up" more highly; a certain proof is to be

This fact of simulation in childhood is often found in the anamneses of neurotics. I have called attention to this phenomenon in the "Psychischen Behandlung der Trigeminus Neuralgie," and have mentioned that children often pretend to be deaf, blind, dumb, etc. E. Jones mentions this fact in his "Hamletstudie," and calls attention to the resemblance of Hamlet's pretense to that of children. There are many historical examples such as Saul, Claudius and others, and they show us the problem in its pure culture. The accompanying thought is always how can I secure myself from a danger, how can I avoid a defeat? It is clear that the neurotic who apperceives according to the analogy man-woman perceives in the domination of a position a masculine equivalent, a substitute and protection for the threatened loss of manliness. And the technique of simulation consists in the fact that the individual sets forth a fiction and acts in accordance therewith as though he had the defect which would require such action, while he knows and maintains that he has no such defect. We maintain that the psychically conditioned neurotic symptom arises in the same way only with this difference that the fiction is not recognized as a fiction, but is held as true.[5]

As is frequently the case, we can obtain the

[5] See theoretical part, Chapter III, "The accentuated fiction."

found in the conduct of small children who throw themselves on the floor angrily and thus try to make themselves dirty in order to attract the attention of their parents, but betray thereby that the idea of "being down" as a fiction of what is forbidden, dirty, sinful, is developing in them. In this psychic gesture of small children may also be detected the model for strongly developed later neurotic traits.

Further notions may be gathered from the impressions of heavenly bodies, as may be seen from a psychological understanding of the various religions and of civilization. The aboriginal races, like the child, regarded the sun, the day, joy, elevation, being "up," as resembling each other and frequently associated "being down" with sin, death, dirt, sickness and night.

The antithesis of "up-down" is not less distinct than in ancient religions. From a work by K. Th. Preuss on "Die Feuergötter als Ausgangspunkt zum Verständniss der Mexicanischen Religion," Mitteilungen der Anthropologischen Gesellschaft in Wien, 1903, we are able to infer the deeply rooted character of this antithesis and the association of "up-down." The fire god is also the god of the dead who live with him at the place of descent.

Overturned vessels, people who fell, were regarded as presentations of "up-downs," that is to say, of falling into the realm of the dead, and thoughts of preservation and destructive activities were given this form of spatial antithesis.[1]

Further, sensations and impressions from childhood tend to give form to the spatial notion of "up-down" and to define the contrast more sharply. Falling, falling down, is painful, blamable, dishonorable, at times, punishable. Not rarely it is the result of inattention, lack of foresight and the child may therefore assume these sensory traces as an admonition, so that being "down" may be felt as a forceful expression for "fallen," for inattention, for unskillfulness, for defeat, not without releasing or at least stimulating the protest which is directed against the approaching feeling of inferiority. In this category of "down-up," one of which cannot be thought of without the other, is further found intermingled trains of thought (in both neurotics and normal persons), which express the antitheses of conquest and defeat, of triumph and inferiority. In individual cases upon analysis memory traces emerge of riding, swimming, flying, mountain climbing, climbing up and of climbing staircases, the antitheses of which reveal themselves as carrying a rider, incubus, sinking in water, falling down, tumbling down, a check

[1] I am especially indebted to Prof. Dr. S. Oppenheim for some important historical data for my work.

in an upward or forward movement. The more abstract and figurative the memory is in dreams, in hallucinations, in separate neurotic symptoms, the more perceptible are the transitions which show a sexual factor. In this connection the masculine principle is only represented by the feeling of greater power, as being "up," and the feminine by the feeling of being "down." It is easy to see that scuffling and its results support this valuation.

In the games of children which are preparatory for the conflicts of life (Karl Groos) this striving "upwards" is regularly found. Also in the thoughts of children concerning a vocation. In the progress of the psychic development reality is seen working as a brake, so that the abstraction "upwards" has a tendency to assume a concrete form in some. Very often in this connection caution in the form of fear of being in elevated positions is at work and changes the wish to be a roof maker into that of being a master builder, makes of the aviator a builder of flying machines, changes the wish of the little girl to be like her father into the more attainable wish of being able to command like her mother.

The striving for security and the masculine protest make the greatest possible use of the resulting guiding lines of the "will to be up." Under the pressure of the fiction the neurotic is sometimes forced to decisions, to conflict and strife, to passionate haste, sometimes to cautious, hesitating, doubting behavior. Thus he is placed in a position to make an estimate of his worth in life and that through instances which escape the notice of others. He must scent out, hold fast, exaggerate or arrange situations which seem to us of very little value. Let us follow this conduct in detail.

A girl, 25 years old, came to us with complaints of frequent headache, emotional attacks, disinclination for life and work. Traces of rickets were perceptible. The history of childhood revealed an extreme feeling of inferiority which was kept at a strained tension because of the mother's preference for a younger brother and because of his intellectual superiority. The most cherished wish of this patient had always been to be big, very wise, and a man. She took the preparatory attitudes for the attainment of this masculine ego-consciousness as far as was possible from her father. When this was not possible for her, a small, stupid girl, she had secured the imaginary ego-consciousness through emotional expedients of rage and anger against her relatives and especially in obstinacy toward her mother, in the simulation of stupidity, of awkwardness and sickness, and finally in the arrangement of laziness. I omit here the lines constructed by her of man-

liness, of malice, of obstinacy, and refrain also
from analyzing her overweening ambition, her
inclination to lying and ostentation, and will content myself with showing how all these habits are
combined in the impulse to be "up" and serve
the tendency to depreciate others.   For this purpose I will refer to one of her dreams, which contains a modest reference to the psychology of
somnambulism.   The dream is as follows:

*"I became a sleepwalker and climbed onto the
head of everybody."*

The patient had heard sleepwalkers spoken of
a few days previous to this dream.   In her attempt at explanation of this dream a series of
ambitious thoughts emerged which takes the
form among others of a sexual picture of domination over her future husband.   She remembered dreams of earlier times which represented
her as riding on a man, on a horse.[2]   I have
never treated a real sleepwalker, but one finds
this neurotic symptom sometimes indicated in on-
sets.   It is manifested as is the dream of flying,
of climbing stairs, etc., as a dynamic expression
of the "will to be up" in the sense of the manly

[2] Women riding on a man one frequently finds as the subject of
paintings.   I wish to call attention to Burgkmair, Hans Baldung,
Grien, Dürer, and to tell of the many prints which show Alexander's paramours riding on Aristotle.

aggression. In a patient who showed strong
masochistic traits, I once discovered strenuous
attempts to reach the ceiling of the room by putting his legs out on the wall during the night.
The interpretation showed that the patient rescued himself from a real or an imagined situation which was regarded as feminine by turning
around to the masculine protest and at the same
time gave expression to this in a symbolic *modus
dicendi* through his striving upwards.

The second thought of the dream, "I climbed
onto the heads of everybody," reveals the same
meaning. The patient makes use here of a form
of speech to express that she is superior to all
others. Her striving upwards is only to be understood dialectically in an antithesis, for the
thoughts of insecure neurotics generally move in
strongly antithetical directions, in an "either-or,"
in an abstraction understood according to the
scheme of the opposites, masculine-feminine.
The innumerable middle ways are not chosen because the two neurotic poles, the feeling of inferiority on the one hand and the overtense ego-
consciousness on the other only permit the
antithetical values to reach consciousness.[3]

[3] That the tentative, insecurely begun, beginnings in philosophy
have likewise hypotasized this antithetical mode of thinking we
have already emphasized.

Karl Joël speaks of this problem in the "Geschichte der Zahl-
prinzipien in der griechischen Philosophie" (Zeitschr. f. Philoso-

The train of thought of this dream permits us to divine the neurotic predispositions of the patient. In reality her masculine protest, her inclination to belittle others, her ambition, her sensitiveness, defiance, unyieldingness, obstinacy, is sufficiently remarkable. The psychic significance of her headache is revealed in this dream. Previous analysis showed in fact that the symptom always made its appearance when there was a feeling of defeat, of belittlement, of emasculation—to speak in the words of the dream, when one "mounted her head." In the phases of the headache, therefore, through the construction of these "expedients of pain" with consequent hallucinations of pain she strove to dominate all persons, especially her mother, and was able to enhance her ego-consciousness thereby in the same manner as she was able to do it through defiance, laziness, and obstinacy, only to a greater degree, in short, had thus mounted on the heads of others.

In children the tendency to be up is unmistakable and coincides with the wish to be big. They wish to be lifted up and like to climb on sofas, tables, boxes, and usually connect with this striving the idea of showing themselves un-

phie und philos. Kritik. Bd. 97), and states in this study, "The real root of 'antithesis' lies in the instinctive, peculiar fixity of thought which only recognizes absolutes."

conquerably courageous, manly. How closely bordering on this is the tendency to depreciate others is shown by their joy when they succeed in being "bigger" than grown people. The heightening of the aggressive tendency is manifested in children who show neurotic symptoms at an early age by this exhibition. Thus it sometimes happens that children in the consulting room of the physician constantly climb on tables and benches and thus reveal their contempt.

The danger of falling, of accidents in striving upwards as well as the customary training to cowardice, force the majority of children to a change of form of the guiding line, or to neurotic, circuitous ways, whereby the fear of elevated positions and heights opposes itself as an admonition usually in a symbolical form to undertakings and ventures of all sorts, and thus becomes the foundation of a predisposition which has the appearance of a neurotic check on aggression. At times the desire to be up is transposed for the most part to a tendency to depreciate others. The tendency of those suffering from dementia præcox to change the furniture stands regularly in such close connection with the depreciation of the surroundings that the suspicion is justified, that this is one of the fictitious, abstract, circuitous ways by which the psychotic enhances his ego-consciousness. In a transferred form this placing of others in an inferior position is expressed in the tendency to calumny, especially, however, in neurotic jealousy and delirium of jealousy. I discovered further an interesting sort of derogation in nervous subjects in their care, their anxious behavior, in their fears for the fate of other people. They act as if others were incapable of caring for themselves without their help. They are constantly giving advice, wish to do everything themselves, are always finding new dangers and are never contented until others confide themselves entirely to their care. Neurotic parents are thus the cause of much harm, and in love and marriage much friction is caused in this manner. One of my patients, who was run over twice in his childhood, associated his feeling of injured personality with this memory and whenever he crossed a street with another person he led that person anxiously over by the arm as though without his help his companion could not have crossed. Many persons are filled with fears when their relatives travel by rail, go swimming or canoeing, give their nurses constant instructions and continue their tendency to depreciation in exaggerated criticisms and corrections. In schools and in offices this nagging depreciation is always found in neurotic teachers and superiors. In the practice of psychotherapy it is one of the main requirements to obviate predispositions of this sort, even when the patient provokes them. This requirement often amounts to a renunciation of authority. Every one who has become acquainted with the hypersensitiveness of neurotic subjects knows with what slight cause they feel themselves to be undervalued. One of my patients who suffered from hystero-epilepsy and always conducted himself as if he wished to place himself in an entirely subordinate position fell on one occasion unconscious before my door. In such "accidents" the tendency to undervaluation is clearly recognizable. While still in a confused condition he addressed me as "Teacher," and stammered that he would bring a note. After the attack he told me that he had come unwillingly on that occasion. The analysis showed that he had come to regard me as a teacher in order to obtain the distance necessary for the conflict, in order to be able to act as though he were obliged to come to the school and to bring a written excuse for his absence. After he had placed himself as far as his feelings were concerned in this situation of inferiority he could allow the compensatory expedients derived therefrom to come into play in order to belittle me.

A girl 20 years old suffered from the compulsory idea that she could not ride in a street-car because when she got in the thought always emerged that a man might get out at the same time and fall under the wheels. Analysis showed that this compulsory neurosis represented the masculine protest of the patient in the figure of being "above" corresponding with which the man must be "under," deprived of value, and should bear the injuries which he imposes on women. In addition the exaggerated striving for security constructed the protection of anxiety which was intended to satisfy further the fear of the male. Even then when her superiority was assured she could not bring herself to decide on marriage, for her future husband would have a hard time with her—from this point of view one is able to understand the often incomprehensible striving of many neurotic girls and women to exact from their partners the greatest sacrifices and put them to the most severe tests, in so far as they hope to attain thereby an enhancement of their ego-consciousness to the point of an appearance of manliness.

Thinking in crude antitheses is therefore in itself a sign of uncertainty and adheres to the sole genuine antithesis, that between male and female. In this a judgment of worth is already given, which infuses itself unnoticed in every "antithesis" (Joel) because this antithesis is always made in the figure of a dissection of the hermaphroditic form into a male and female half.

Plato has perhaps expressed this idea most
purely. And human perception was unable until
the time of Kant to disentangle itself from this
self-made fiction. But the neurotically disposed
child adheres to the oppositeness of the sexes and
to the higher valuation of the male principle
therewith connected in order to escape from uncertainty and in order to find a guiding line for
his idea of egoistic worth. Thus it happens that
this guiding fiction contains a manly aspect, and
that in all the experiences and strivings of neurotic individuals the masculine protest is revealed
as the ordering principle and motive force. The
antithesis of the sexes is admirably expressed in
the above given symbol of the spatial opposites of
"up-down." And thus it becomes comprehensible that in every one of our psychological analyses
this expression of a sharp antithetical schema
must somehow or other come to light. It is still
an open question whether reënforcements of the
antithesis have been acquired from the events of
early childhood and the resulting impressions,
from the observations of sexual relations in human beings and animals, or whether the consciousness of the higher position of the male has
been fixed by the normal situations of sexual relations.

The "will to be above" of the neurotic woman
is produced by her manly guiding idea and repre-

sents an attempt to identify herself with the man.
The importunity and rigidity with which this
takes place even in neurotic, circuitous ways testi-
fies to the original uncertainty and fear of being
"below," undervalued, female. Thus the transcendental egoistic idea attains its powerful
dominancy because it promises compensation, the
overcoming of the feeling of inferiority, in the
opposite direction. Every gesture then says, "I
will be above, I will be a man because I am afraid
as a woman of being oppressed and misused."
Ambition and envy are hereby strengthened and
an unusually lively mistrust is awakened against
every possibility of belittlement. Where there
is real undervaluation, however, the masculine
protest flashes forth and leads from slight and
often from no cause to the well known, unpleasant frictions of the neurotic individual with his
environment, in which the principal weapons of
attack used to confirm the feeling of power are
disputatiousness, love for justice, obstinate adherence to opinion and trust in penetration.
And in this connection the tendency to "look beneath" will never be absent, especially in times
of uncertainty, the acute perception of affronts,
neglects, undervaluations, and further than this
arrangements of depression, anxiety, remorse,
feeling of guilt and pangs of conscience.
Stronger measures for security are applied and

new neurotic symptoms and deviations are constructed, the neurotic traits of character become more deeply seated and more abstract and the fully developed picture of the neurosis arises.[4] Thus the revolt for attaining a heightened ego-consciousness is fairly contrived, the introduction thereof is formed by the disease itself and by the predispositions to disease which in some way or other are made use of as means for attaining power in the environment.

A patient, 21 years old, came under treatment because of extreme depression, loss of sleep and compulsory thoughts. It was ascertained that she had always had neurotic traits of character.

[4] While writing this book I discovered in Alfred v. Berger's "Hofrat Eysenhardt" an excellent example of the type just described in whom the striving to be above was especially well marked and whose lectures I would recommend to every psychotherapeutist. One will find in this description a repetition of all we have said concerning this type of individual from a poet's standpoint. The all too powerful *elan* of the father, the feeling of inferiority of the boy along with the compensatory masculine protest. The accentuation of sexual desire, of the will to power, the preparation for the patricide, fetichism, contentious tendency, the exaggerated assurance in the case of threatening defeat. The construction of remorse, self-reproach, hallucinations, and compulsory ideas as a revengeful annihilation of the authority of the State. The loss of a tooth and the exaggerated fear of woman as the result of a further accentuated masculine protest, and along with this the repeated arrangement of an exaggerated sexual desire, all of which is very impressive and obvious, a description of the neurotic subterfuge which reminds one of Dostoyeffsky's descriptions and which requires no further elucidation.

The compulsory neurosis broke out as her relations with a man whom she wanted to marry became serious.   The typical pathogenic situation brings the neurotic "no" to light, and while the patient was making her preparations for marriage, and did not hesitate with the affirmative answer, she arranged for the neurosis and conducted herself as if she did not wish to marry. In all these very numerous cases the next step is a condition which therefore takes the form, "If I were well, if I should overcome my present condition," etc. (in men, often: "If I were potent"), "I would marry."   By this condition, which is equivalent to a vacillation, a doubt, to a special attitude of caution, the patient escapes all responsibility, has drawn the bolt in secret until something further happens, but may act as if he wishes to open the door.   The traits of mistrust, of disputatiousness, of tyranny, and of wishing to be "above" are clearly revealed in the analysis, and one can easily comprehend that the fear of not being equal to the partner, the menace of feeling another superior in love or marriage necessitates the secret retreat and constructs the neurotic symptom.   Not rarely one finds a purposeful valuation of the person's own sexuality from which without proof or with the assistance of memories which every one has at command, or by evoking unconscious falsifications the impression is sought that it is too little or too great to permit a marriage to be ventured on.

The further communication of the patient explained that she could undertake nothing because whenever she began anything the thought emerged that it was useless because every one must die. As one sees, a nonsensical thought, which at the same time has sense, but above all brings time and development to a standstill and renders the entrance of the patient upon marriage impossible. In accordance with this the conviction that the patient only came to the physician because she was forced to, that she had no hope of cure and only desired proof of her incurability followed as a matter of course. One of her dreams showed much of this constellation. It was as follows:

"A physician came to me who said I should jump and sing when thoughts of death came to me, then the thoughts would vanish. Then a child (hesitatingly), a large one is brought. It had pain and cried. It was given medicine so that it should become quiet and sleep."

The physician in the dream had once treated her as a child when she had scarlet fever. In the dream he used the words which she during her present illness had constantly heard from her

relatives and from physicians. He gives her advice of a kind which amounts to nothing. These
thoughts are aimed at me and express the conviction that all my measures will be useless. Of
course this dream was dreamed during a night
when she slept—for the first time after a period
of insomnia. As the patient, however, saw in
this fact a partial success of the treatment she
realized with strong aggression my measures too
were useless. The hesitation in emphasizing the
"largeness" of the child shows on what the
thoughts of the dreamer are dwelling, on a small,
a newborn child. The expression, "a child is
brought" (supply: into the world) is taken from
the idea of giving birth and coincides with this
in the outlined representation of the dream. The
powder which is given to the child is the sleeping
powder of the patient in a former treatment, an
indication that pains also belong to the patient,
to giving birth. In other words the patient here
expresses: I cannot sleep because I think of giving birth with its pains. Giving birth, pains,
dying, in these she sees her fate and hence
she thinks of dying in order to avoid giving
birth.

The exaggerated security against childbirth is
a change of form and intensity of her masculine
protest. In order to secure herself against the
feminine rôle she enters upon the neurotic devi-

ation, fixes her thought upon an anticipatory tendency on childbirth and death as admonitions and prefers to become a child, to take a powder rather than to be cured psychotherapeutically. Because her cure signifies her fitting herself into the feminine rôle. Now the conflict is turned more acutely against the physician who wishes to cure her insomnia. She must remain superior to him, must permit him to talk absurdities and dictate to him, that he should treat her with medicines as she had been treated when a child. The compulsory neurosis represents her reassuring philosophy of the vanity of everything under the sun.

In our sort of neuropsychology one always gains the impression that the visible neurotic conduct is directed straight to the final purpose, to the fictitious goal, as if one were examining one of the intermediary pictures in a cinematographic film. The problem consists in recognizing this conduct, that is, the symptoms, predispositions, and traits of character, and to learn to comprehend their object. In every neurotic attitude the beginning and final purpose is concealed in its significance.[5] These facts form the foundation

[5] Bergson justly emphasizes the same thing for every move of life. One who possesses sufficient insight and experience is able to see in every psychic phenomenon the past, present, and future, but also the desired finale. Thus every psychic phenomenon and every trait of character, similarly to the inferior somatic

of every individualistic psychological method and coincide with our other findings. Therefore in the analysis of a symptom or of a dream the feeling of effeminacy, of inferiority, of being "down," and the masculine protest, the fictitious manly goal, the feeling of being "above," will always be found indicated, in the form of an upwardly directed psychic attitude, in a hermaphroditic picture which is apperceived in a strongly antithetical manner, in neurotic, circuitous ways, which as such characterize the tendency to meet obstacles with expedients, or when analyzed reveal at one time the tendency upwards, at another the tendency downwards in the alterations and vacillations of the psychic phenomena. Frequently this "will to be up" is expressed in a strongly figurative manner, especially in dreams, but also in symptoms, and takes the symbolic form of a race, of soaring, of climbing mountains, of emerging from water, etc., while the "down" is represented by falling, in short by a motion downwards. Just as frequently the figure or the fact of the sexual act is symbolically employed for the same expression. I will here give an account of the dreams of a patient who had fears for his future as a man on account of his weakness and noticeably effeminate conduct. In a

organ, is to be looked upon as a symbol of life, as an attempt at an ascendancy of the masculine protest.

dream of his early childhood which for a long time filled him with fears he saw himself pursued by a bull. As a farmer's son he understood at that early age that the male pursuer represented a race for a cow, that is, for the patient himself. When he was to enter school he directed his steps straight to the girls' school and had to be taken to the boys' school by force. He unconsciously regarded his life as a race, for which he constantly found preparations. When he was courting a girl his friend cut him out. When he contemplated marriage, he became afraid of the superiority of his wife, fell into the habit of compulsory masturbation, suffered from frequent pollutions, and fell victim to a tremor, which hindered his work and advancement in office. Naturally he set up the condition that he would only marry when he was cured, a thought which seemed to be wise and justified, but which permitted the patient to operate secretly against his marriage as behind a veil because he feared therefrom a reduction of his ego-consciousness. The tremor represented to him the premonitions of a paralysis which he feared on account of his excessive masturbation. After he had secured himself in this manner he still felt the need of confirmation of his incurability and went weeping to physicians. Our conversation revealed to me the picture of a restless, ambitious individual who wished constantly to detract from others, but who recoiled in fear from a serious decision. Amorous relations were also with him principally a means of assuring himself of his superior manliness. No matter how eagerly he courted a girl, the moment she met his addresses, she lost all charm for him. Besides as soon as he approached an engagement he entered into other relations without prospect, or gave them a prospectless form and thus ran after his rejections in order to be able through the feeling of his lack of influence even vis-a-vis his future bride, to be able to regard himself as inferior. From this he constantly regained the impulse to work secretly against the apparently desired marriage. One of his dreams is as follows:

"I was with my old friend and was speaking with him about a mutual friend. He said, 'Of what use is his money to him, he has learned nothing?'"

The old friend, who had cut our patient out in the courtship of a girl, had failed in the Technical school and had given up study. The patient was superior to him for he had finished the course. He embraced the sublime principle, "Knowledge is more than money," especially as this profession served his fiction to be "above" and comforted him. The mutual acquaintance is placed here instead of the rich girl who was courted by both. The contest begins anew. Our patient is declared victor by his rival.

A second dream which occurred the same night makes this clearer. The patient dreamed:

"As if I had caused the fall of a girl of lower standing and had dishonored her."

The fiction of this dream says a shade more clearly that he is "above." The girl who was formerly courted is thus in the sense of the patient brought down, made poor, and recognizes him as her master.

I will here briefly mention that the occurrence of several dreams in a night signifies that various attempts at preliminary arrangements of tentative solutions of a problem are undertaken. It becomes regularly apparent that a single way is not sufficient for the guiding, egoistic idea of caution, a fact which is easily comprehended in the case of neurotics. The dream then, under the influence of the more intensive craving for security becomes more abstract, more figurative, and one thus obtains in interpreting all the dreams of a night several psychic attitudes, from the comparison of which the dynamic of the neurosis becomes much clearer. In the above cited case the rival surrenders and the wealth of the girl—her power—is deprived of worth for him. The second dream deprives the girl also of power and places her in the position a woman that is "under" occupies, and this is done in the most far-fetched and abstract manner, so that nothing personal is left to the girl under consideration except her subordinate position.   The patient besides expresses the thought that only an uneducated girl from the country serves his purpose, as he can always remain her master.   The girl whom he wishes to make his wife frightens him because of her intelligence.[6]   This is the tendency of many neurotics, which causes them always to choose below their social level, and thus thoughts and facts come to pass such as choosing a prostitute or a little girl for love and marriage, necrophilic tendencies, etc.   In all similar cases the tendency to detract from the partner is perceptible, which seeks to degrade the wife by the construction of mistrust, jealousy, tyranny, ethical principles and requirements.

A further idea shown in a dream represents a race graphically:

"I was riding in a railway car and looked out of the window to see if the dog was still running with the train.   I thought that he had run himself to death, had fallen under the wheels.   I felt

[6] Another dream of the same night may have dealt with the violation of a girl.

sorry for him.   Then the idea struck me that I had another dog, but a clumsy one."

He had often ridden bicycle races with his old friend and rival and was usually left behind. Now as his friend occupies a position socially inferior to him, his friend "can run after him," as one says in Vienna when a person gives himself airs.   The metamorphosis into a dog is a product of the tendency to derogation and is quite frequently met with.   In a case of dementia precox I observed that the patient gave all dogs the names of women of importance.   The dog also represented his future bride who also brought his superiority into question.   Her death, moreover, would free him of his fear, just as he would also be free if she should listen to another suitor, as his suspicion often whispered to him was the case.   "If she should fall under the wheels."   "If this should occur, it would cause him sorrow." In the dream he regards this as having already happened and anticipates his sorrow.   The "clumsy dog" is a girl who about this time had disgusted him by meeting his advances and for whom he no longer cared.

His dislike for those above him is boundless and deep-seated.   One night he dreamed:

"Our singing society gave a concert.   The director's place was empty."

The society to which he belonged was on one occasion obliged to sing without a director because the latter had missed the train. This situation appeared to him better than any other. "We need no director," he thought. This is his usual attitude in all situations in which he himself is not the director.

The impulse to masturbation in male neurotics corresponds in female neurotics to the tendency to avoid a decision and thereby to remain "up." In the masturbation phantasies of girls the woman is often found to take the rôle of a man. Also the position which is taken therein is at times that of the man. In men masturbation serves, first, as proof that one can live alone, second, as a protection against and hindrance to sexual relations which on account of the superiority of the wife are feared and hence arises from the craving for security. If the situation necessitates stronger securities, impotence or the developed neurosis makes its appearance, not as a consequence of renunciation of masturbation, but as a reënforced security. The masturbation phantasies in neurotics have often a masochistic or sadistic feature, according to the phase of the masculine protest which they aim to represent.

Among the preparatory actions and neurotic expedients which are intended to serve to secure the position of being "up," curiosity, impulse to investigation, the desire to see everything, the "voyeur" impulse mentioned by writers occupies a prominent place. These impulses are always a proof of a primary uncertainty for the compensation of which the guiding lines of investigation are brought in. They serve especially in developed neuroses secondarily the purposes of dilatoriness to avoid a plan and a decision and are in life, especially in the erotic very often changed from a means to an end on which all the psychic activities are based. Investigation, the search for truth, the wish to understand everything, the well known neurotic thoroughness, these are then the traits which the ego-consciousness erects and must elevate or protect.

CHAPTER VII

PUNCTUALITY, THE WILL TO BE FIRST, HOMOSEX-
UALITY AND PERVERSION AS A SYMBOL, MOD-
ESTY AND EXHIBITIONISM, CONSTANCY AND
INCONSTANCY, JEALOUSY

A PHENOMENON often noted in neurotics is
their attitude towards the question of punctuality.
In accordance with our analysis of neurotic
pedantry the expectation is justified that a large
number of punctual individuals will be found
among neurotics. This is in fact the case. But
it is easy to perceive that these patients play with
the thought, how would it be if they should let
others wait, a train of thought which indicates
their opposition to others. There always remains in this attitude of punctuality so much of
aggression that these patients exact the greatest
punctuality from everybody without exception
and in consequence are often in a position to put
their expedients and neurotic preparedness to
attacks into operation at the tardiness of others.
In other cases it is found that pride compels them
to come late regularly, and when others are
obliged to wait and a flood of excuses is offered,

this is felt as an enhancement of the ego-consciousness. This tardiness is well fitted to form a substitute for the fear of decisions. The social fitness is greatly menaced and professional duties as well as relations with friends and loved ones are soon eliminated. Admonitions are entirely fruitless, because the obstinate attitude is only confirmed by them. The neurotic is able to master the situation by his eternal tardiness and thus place before his relatives an insoluble problem. The choice of this line of character often follows in conformity with an analogy: "as I came into the world too late among my brothers and sisters," "because I did not arrive later like my younger brother or sister." It may be seen from this how, by this neurotic arrangement—the feeling of inferiority and the order of birth of the brothers and sisters—a broad and permanent basis of operation for the battle for superiority is gained. Patients who always come too early show also at other times the trait of impatience. Through a feeling of inferiority they are constantly in fear of other new losses and reassure themselves by believing in their "unlucky star." In cases of these neurotics, too, the elder brother is often found as an opponent with whom they are engaged, as it were, in a race, an analogical fiction, but by no manner of means the causal factor of their conduct.

Fictive rights of primogeniture become often for younger children the impetus for the enhancement of the egoistic idea, and in my experience second and later children show greater tendency to neuroses and psychoses, and certainly show greater ambition.[1]   In their neurotic conduct the figurative analogy of the story of Jacob and Esau comes to light, proving that the wish to be first is at the foundation of the situation.   Their preparations and predispositions will always have as object to permit no one to have merit, to transform every relation by means of love and hate so that their superiority shall become apparent.   The tendency to derogation exceeds all bounds.   The individual of this type does not hesitate at harming himself if he can only harm others at the same time.   In the formal change of the guiding line a view such as Cæsar took is often arrived at, "Better first in a village than second in Rome," better to play the leading rôle with the mother or father than to draw an unknown lottery ticket in marriage, etc.   Hatred is frequently felt for superiors, teachers and physicians.   They are usually kill-joys in social gatherings, as soon as their superiority is not recognized and they often break off every relation of friendship and love after a short time, if the

[1] Compare Frischauf, "The Psychology of the Younger Brother," E. Reinhardt, Munich (in preparation).

other parties to these relationships do not acknowledge themselves inferior. Very often their conduct is brusque and inimical from the start, because they are already at strife before the other person suspects it. They cannot endure to have any one stand or walk before them, and avoid every school examination, because the superiority of the person conducting the examination is unendurable to them. That all these phenomena may finally be directed against the family environment, and take the form of the view that the family must care for the patient is a further step towards the proof of the significance and importance of the egoistic idea for the patient. At times they operate with their neuroses as others carry on fortune hunting.

Frequently the wish to be first, with the wife, is hidden in the neurotic efforts of a male patient and he hunts through her previous life with jealousy and suspicion and constantly believes himself deceived, or he eagerly keeps watch lest his wife should prefer another, the fear of the wife as the expression of the feeling of incomplete manliness. The neurotic only wants certainty in regard to this point and even goes so far as to put the wife to all sorts of tests. In the burning jealousy which from this point on possesses the neurotic the expedients by which the wife is degraded follow of themselves and the egoistic feeling of the jealous neurotic is thereby so greatly elevated that he is often not in a condition to separate from the justly or unjustly accused person. This latter fact which is often met with is wholly dependent on the masculine guiding idea of the patient. He cannot endure the thought that one could abandon him and reconstructs the facts in such a way that he is hindered, by love, by pity, by fear of misfortune which might come to wife or children from taking the final step.

Perhaps the striving to be first, to be master of all, is constructed on a feeling of inferiority based with justification or without it on smallness of stature or of the genital organs. In the developed neurosis the patient through the arrangement of a neurotic symptom fails at a distance from the opportunity in which he was to have given proof. As a frequent symptom of this sort I was able to observe compulsory blushing.

In a less marked degree the tendency to be first is a universal human characteristic and concomitant therewith is regularly found an inclination to conflict in all human beings. The competitive race begins even in earliest childhood and creates its psychic organs and reassuring traits of character. Thus one often finds in children the trait of character that they wish to be the first to eat or drink or that they like to run ahead in order to reach a place before others.

Not rarely at five years of age they carry on the play of trying to outrun every wagon and many child's games owe their origin to the idea of competitive races. Many persons preserve this inclination throughout their entire life in the form of an unconscious gesture, always wish to walk at the head in a company or hasten their steps when any one attempts to pass them on the street. In a transferred sense this tendency makes itself noticeable by the fact that those who possess it are given to hero-worship whereby the more profound sense comes to light of being himself, also Heros, Achilles, Alexander, Hannibal, Cæsar, Napoleon or Archimedes, and thus betraying at the same time the guiding fiction and the original feeling of inferiority. The likeness to God also reveals itself as an active fiction and is manifested at times in fairy tales, in phantasy, and in the psychoses. We have emphasized that in this state of the predispositions and traits of character all bonds of friendship and love are threatened and when the stronger uncertainty requires it, forces the patient into doubt, makes him represent scarecrows or ideal forms by means of which he secures himself permanently from reality. A caricature of Cæsar, he now seeks his mother, the small city, the lower relations, wanders at times restlessly from one place of residence to another as if the external relations were the cause of his dissatisfaction. In this developed neurosis the sexual appetite is frequently directed to children, persons of low station, maids; homosexuality, perverse inclinations or inclinations to masturbation are constructed and adhered to because the patient hopes thus more easily to master the situation. For the fear of a woman hinders a natural sexual relation to such an extent that the neurotic in order to avoid the defeat of which he stands in fear, arrives at the expedient of *ejaculatio precox,* of pollutions, and of impotence.

The circumstances are similar in neurotic women of this type, in whom frequently rivalry in society with friends in the large city, with sisters, with a daughter and a daughter-in-law is secretly brewing, forces to neurotic securities and this causes illness. In male neurotics the social position leads to the development of a neurosis as soon as precedence in society, in science or in amusement is called into question and contested.

Where the feeling of inferiority of the younger child forms the fictitious guiding ideal according to the pattern of the first born or the earliest born the most varied real and apparent advantages incite the desire and envy of the younger child. Nearly always teachers will notice traits such as envy of the size of the older brother, of his growth of hair, of the size of his genital organs. That fictitious values are thereto given I was able to infer from the psychotherapeutic treatment of two brothers, of whom each had envied the other in childhood on account of the development of the genital organs. In the same manner the real preference of the elder brother or such as arises naturally from the situation becomes the point of attack. The fact that he is taken to the theater and on journeys, that he has more experience in the sexual problem, is sexually active, that he is preferred by girls and by the servants may fill the younger child, where there is a feeling of inferiority, with the most profound bitterness. For this melancholy, at times a hopeless emotional condition, arose at a very early age in our patient and attained an incredible degree. At times there seems no prospect of victory in the competition. His manly tendency turns around toward the pseudomasochistic side [2] and seeks now to attain the manly goal by emphasizing the feelings of sickness and weakness, by yielding and submitting to an extreme degree in the hope of thus winning the protection of parents and those with more strength and to gain in this manner the desired security in life. I have seen cases

[2] According to our conception, every perversion and inversion is a simile, a symbol. For pseudomasochism see "The Psychic Treatment of Trigeminal Neuralgia," l. c.

where protracted catarrh in childhood (Czerny's exudative diathesis) was sustained by a combination of the clearing of the throat and panting and led to sneezing fits and asthma (see Strümpell's Asthma-theory) and in connection with which at the same time fictions of pregnancy and castration and exaggerated anal sensitiveness effected a homosexual factor which was to be understood symbolically. In one of these cases the fictitious feminine presentation went so far that the patient came to identify himself with his younger sister by a change of form of the guiding line. And as the mother showed a noticeable inclination always to be late, he took this fact and the wish that he had been born later in place of his younger sister as a guiding motive always to arrive late wherever he went, even when he came to me for treatment, a phenomenon which did not vanish when it was revealed, but only after a cure had been effected. In these feminine presentations the masculine protest is striven after by a circuitous route, by following the feminine guiding line and is regularly accompanied by day dreams, sensitiveness, disputatiousness, discontent, and is also as a rule forced into side paths by fear of tests, of decisions, of the sexual partner, so that perverse tendencies, onanism and pollutions are frequently found. The initial phenomena of inferiority of organs may disappear or only remain as a trace. Smallness and anomalies of the exterior genital organs may sometimes be discovered, but as a rule only reveal themselves psychically in the fear of not being able to dominate the sexual partner. This emotional condition often leads to jealousy, tendency to torment and sadistic inclinations, by which it is sought to establish the proof of potency and of being loved.

Often the pride of the patient is so great that he is himself not conscious of his jealousy. According to our experience the solution of this psychic constellation is that the masculine protest in addition to other effects has also the effect of repressing jealousy in order to prevent a diminution of personal worth. The consequence of this repression is not great, at most that the patient finds himself in ambiguous situations. Generally he acts as if he were jealous and often so plainly that every one else except the patient knows it. At times, however, the jealousy is masked by depression, headache, refuge in solitude, etc.

I will give still another dream of a patient who came under my treatment because of depression and anxiety in society, because in the partial interpretations undertaken by the patient this dream reveals many of the points just described of the competition of a neurotic with his older brother:

"*It seemed to me that I had made a bet with my brother Joseph to beat him to a certain place which was not distinguishable in the dream.*

"*I saw myself now suddenly in a little three-wheeled automobile on the road, and tried to direct the automobile as well as possible by means of a small apparatus similar to a key which I was only able to take between the thumb and index finger. I rode very insecurely and felt uncomfortable. I got into by-paths on which I could go no farther. The people whom I met were astonished and laughed. I was forced to take the auto on my back and turn back to the road. There I rode farther in the same manner.*

"*Suddenly I saw myself with my three-wheeled vehicle in the room of an inn which was well known to me and was situated on a mountain near my native place. I now shoved my automobile into a corner and troubled myself no more about it. My brother had arrived before me at the same inn and alongside there was sitting a well-known family who were deeply in debt, consisting of Mr. and Mrs. M—— and their two daughters. My brother and I paid no attention to them. Then Mr. M—— came to our table, spoke with us, and finally we went to the table of the family which, however, was unpleasant to me.*

"The thought of a bet came up in the course of a conversation with my brother. He advised me not to bind myself at an early age to the flighty girl that I wished to marry and told me from his own experiences what ill results this can have to a man striving for success. I comprehended this and promised to act according to his advice. He took little stock in such promises. That incited me to a bet. In early years before I knew what lay buried in the depths of his nature he seemed to be a model to me and I strove to become like him in character, mode of thought, and bearing. Now I see, that I must not pattern after him in many things, if I do not wish to follow in his footsteps.

"It is easier to reach one's destination with an automobile than on foot. This auto, however, obviously represented the wife, to whom I had tied myself. A three-wheeled auto is less perfect than a four-wheeled one, the former lacks something. Thus it is with a woman. Man is perfect. For that reason the antithesis, the small handle. In my earliest youth I was constantly seeking after something in girls. There was something I could not understand about them. Frequently we were led to go under a bridge and yet we did not know what we expected to see through the cracks above.   At that time—I was perhaps five years old—I had not the slightest idea of sexual procedures ('uncertainty') and had also come upon no sexual aberration.   I can, however, say that even at that time something drew me to girls, 'the small handle on the auto' indicated at the same time that I possessed a too small penis or none at all, for which reason the girl must be superior to me.

"I came into by-paths with my auto, that is, through the woman, through which I could not pass and which brought me no nearer to the goal which I wished to attain, that is, no nearer to the summit of my efforts.

"I took the auto on my back—the woman was thus more than ever above me.

"The inn in which I finally found myself with my brother stood on the top of a mountain, this signified my burning desire for success in life, as I had expected it of my brother.

"That I met with a family which was deeply in debt indicates that I had often had exaggerated thoughts concerning the cost of a wife to her husband and that the wife is too often the cause of running into debt.

"It is clear to me also that trains of thought on masturbation (by-paths, being in debt) run through the dream, as well as the false connection of masturbation and the stunting of the genitals.   The latter I ascribe to my uncertainty in regard to my bride.   Without knowing it I hit upon all sorts of expedients for getting rid of her (in the corner).   My condition of depression serves the same purpose, to be liberated from my wife, to prove my superiority in life."

In our physiognomic of the soul we understand the theory of character to be this, we have already frequently spoken of those obvious and deep-seated wants which seek to support and maximate the ego-consciousness as an obtrusive proof of manliness, as if there were a constant fear of becoming "de-classed," of the revelation of a feminine rôle.   Thus the exaggerated modesty of many neurotics, who can visit no public toilet, who suffer from inhibition of the flow of urine in the presence of others, who withdraw from female society on account of blushing or anxiety and palpitation of the heart, reveals to us the strained manly ambition, which supports itself against the original feeling of inferiority. The masculine protest of these patients, insecure to the core, forces them to this arrangement whose boundaries pass over into those of bashfulness and awkwardness: or there is a concordance of these and other traits which may on occasion supplant each other.   Often in neurotic persons of both sexes one finds an inability to go to the toilet in cases of great necessity before others. The greater modesty of women, especially of neurotic women, in all relations of life originates from the fear which is implanted in them from earliest childhood that attention might be directed to their sex. I have often convinced myself that the performances of girls and women suffer considerably from this more or less unconscious impression, indeed that the progress in the mental development—just as is the case in male patients, who feel unmanly—the formation of social and professional relations and relations of love are immediately checked as soon as the patient comes into a "feminine" or subordinate rôle or presupposes this expectation in others.

This fact is in no manner affected when expressed or repressed sexual stimuli come to light as the apparent source of the checks of aggression. They are similarly arranged, have the purpose of enhancing the fear of the partner and of permitting the retreat decided upon in the plan of life to be entered upon with certainty, are therefore also acts of foresight. The neurotic had already in childhood laid the foundation of this foresight and in it is reflected the feeling of shame as the guiding line of reassuring modesty and the prudery of civilization. The previous history of the patient reveals the exaggerated modesty and this is true at times of those who in

other respects show a boyish nature, and the anxiety of nervous children on being exposed may be
observed in their conduct. They exclude every
one from the room and will lock the doors when
they are going to undress. This conduct is also
often observed in boys who have grown up among
girls. The masculine protest of the latter is expressed in these cases in the derogation of the
boy, either purposely or unthinkingly until he
goes so far as to hide his sex. For the development of the neuroses this expedient of cowardice
has an unfavorable significance. It is equal to
later castration thoughts and wishes of the neurotic, wishes to be a woman, as soon as the fear
of the wife seems actual, or as soon as he wishes
to escape a decision. And it arises nevertheless
originally from the compulsion of an exaggerated
masculine protest, which is easily perceptible
from the accompanying, often continuing traits
of character, such as tyranny, burning ambition,
the desire to have everything, to be first everywhere; from the emotional predispositions to
rage and anger and finally from the tendency to
derogate and to too great foresight.

If therefore neurotic modesty should be considered equal to the secret attempt to play the
man, this "consciousness of rôle" (Groos) is more
clearly manifested in the apparently antithetical
trait of character of shamelessness. In reality

this latter line proves to be a reënforcement and continuation of the former, as an obtrusive reminder to the environment that one is a man. The guiding idea, which causes the predisposition to or habit of exhibitionistic gestures, hence often insulting or tactless obtrusion in respect to the environment betrays in detail the strong masculine factor.   Thus it is when in nervous boys and men sexual exhibitionism breaks through or is expressed habitually in certain faults of toilette. In all similar cases one finds the belief in the power of the phallus constructed as in the antique religious cults as consciousness of power. Narcissistic traits are also regularly intermingled so that in these cases the attitude of conquest, accompanied by coquetry, by the inability to believe in a refusal, attracts the attention.   In shameless girls the trait is even more noticeable because it is unusual.   In conversation, in dress, in behavior, at times only in small things, at times obscurely or in coprology they demonstrate their inability to adapt themselves to or to satisfy themselves with their feminine rôle.   The basis of operation for both sexes is manifested then in such a way that each demands from the other recognition or an extreme submission.   In the analysis of such neurotic girls, at times only in their dreams and symptoms is observed the childish expectation of a metamorphosis into a male

and in other cases always as an attempted substitute for the will to power, the wish to be above.
If two persons of this sort meet, the result is not
rarely that the reënforced masculine guiding line
of the one affects the other preliminarily as a
sort of miracle, a talisman, because in her guiding
ideal the belief in the miraculousness and wonder
working power of manliness is also contained.
Thus there is often for both what seems a chance
fulfilling of destiny, but which is really brought
about by the power of their idea of personality.
One often finds immodest conduct in neurotic
girls as an anticipation of their fictitious expectation; they conduct themselves as if they were
really a boy or a man, expose themselves naked
or live out in neurotic symptoms, dreams and
phantasies their masculine reincarnation.   Often
in such patients the attempt is observed to ascribe
the miraculous power of the phallus by means of
an alteration of form of the fiction to other parts
of the body, for example to the hands, feet,
breasts, which thus altered into male members are
taken into especial favor as fetiches and enjoy a
Narcissus-form worship, as often also the genital
organs or the whole body.   This fetichism is
nearly always transferred to the articles of clothing and constitutes a large part of the charm of
fashion, from which we therefore must assume
that this, like the fetichism itself, must be re-

garded as a substitute of manliness with its larger sphere of usefulness, which has been lost but which is always to be sought.

Like immodesty the deep-seated neurotic infidelity of many sick patients is an imitation of the exaggerated, apperceived masculine image. It indicates to us one of the ways which the masculine goal is forced to take. It is, like many of the neurotic traits of character, often only ideal, a maker of humor or of the view of life (Marczinowsky) or extends only to the boundary where the reality of the female rôle begins. Much oftener the virtue of fidelity is chosen as the means of security in the fear of the man. Phantasies of infidelity, at times to the degree of hallucinations or dreams, often result where there is real or imagined subjection exacted by the husband. Phantasies of prostitution indicate in these cases the neurotic, exaggerated perspective concerning the power of the sexual appetite and serve the same purpose of gaining security. In general in patients who are prone to speak of their sexuality the suspicion is justified that they paint their bugbear with great exaggeration. The reality is always in their favor. In girls often the holy conviction of their infidelity occupies the foreground entirely. It may be therefrom inferred that for them even a single man would be too much and that they wish to protect themselves from love and especially from marriage: "for where does my passion drive me?" The real infidelity of many persons, too, both men and women, is the result of the fear of the partner of whose superiority they are afraid. The understanding of the accompanying symptoms, fear of solitude, fear of places, fear of society, etc., unsocial conduct, fixation of faults of childhood and derogation of the opposite sex are other signs by which the masculine purpose of these traits of character is revealed. Often despised love gives rise to a feeling of a reduction of the egoistic sense to such a degree that hate, indifference or infidelity are the forms which the masculine protest assumes.

In this place a few educational observations may be added, which I was in a position to make in regard to neurotics suffering from jealousy. They all have reference to the search for proofs of the influence of the individual over the partner and every situation which is even half-way fitted for this purpose is made use of. The insatiableness with which the neurotic tests his partner is an indication of the want of self-confidence, of his lack of self-esteem, of his uncertainty so that it is easy to be seen how his jealous efforts serve to bring him more into notice, to attract more attention to himself and thus to secure his self-esteem. The old feeling of being disregarded and neglected is seen to be revived upon the slightest occasion together with the childish attitude of wishing to have everything, to obtain a proof of superiority from the partner. A glance, a word in company, an acknowledgment of a favor, a show of sympathy for a picture, for an author, for a relative, even a protective attitude towards servants may be taken as the cause of the operation. In severe cases the impression is distinctly given that the jealous individual cannot rest because he has no confidence in peaceful happiness on account of his misfortune. Now the neurosis develops in which the effort is made to bend the partner by an arrangement of attacks, to arouse the sympathy of the partner, or the attack is intended as a punishment. Headaches, weeping fits, conditions of weakness, paralysis, attacks of anxiety and depression, silence, etc., have the same value as abandoment to alcoholism, masturbation, perversion and lewdness. The lines of distrust and doubt—often about the legitimacy of the children—become more pronounced, outbreaks of wrath and scolding, mistrust of the entire opposite sex are regular phenomena and reveal the other side of jealousy as a preparation for the derogation of the other. Often pride prevents consciousness of jealousy; the conduct is the same. The situation is not rarely made worse by the circumstance that the other party meets the helplessness of the jealous person with an unconscious satisfaction, thereby giving foundation to his feeling of superiority and does not therefore find the right tone, the proper attitude to hold the jealousy at least within limits. Jealousy of children often leads to grave faults of education. The belief in miracles as a threat to the sexual organs through births or aging nearly always causes jealous excitement to be more strongly manifested in neurotically disposed persons.

CHAPTER VIII

FEAR OF THE PARTNER; THE IDEAL IN THE NEU-
ROSIS; INSOMNIA AND COMPULSION TO SLEEP;
NEUROTIC COMPARISON OF MAN AND WOMAN;
FORMS OF THE FEAR OF THE WIFE

In this striving of the neurotic for the attainment of the masculine guiding goal, one never
misses the fact, as has already been emphasized,
that the fear of a decision resolves itself into a
fear of the opposite sex, that touchstone of the
individual's own power, the fulfiller of the guiding idea. One finds in the family life of boys
and girls, in their play and phantasy, in their
assortment of experiences of all kinds, in their
day dreams and poems and in their living out
of actual experiences preparations for the struggle for supremacy so early, with such abundance
and such unity of purpose that in arriving at
puberty secure determinants for love and marriage already exist and by these alone the choice
and direction of their eroticism is defined within
narrow limits. Let us consider now of what nature these determinants of love objects may be
in neurotics. Among these should be mentioned

tyranny, hypersensitiveness, ambition, discontent and all the principal neurotic character-traits already described, the security-giving devices of mistrust, caution, jealousy and derogatory tendency which is everywhere seeking faults, the neurotic digressions and subterfuges which are at first directed against members of their own family, and which are intended, with this as a basis, to prove their own superiority or to facilitate the escape of the superiority of others. The neurotic device has its part in this and demands for love some quality which is difficult of attainment or entirely out of reach, or that the sexual partner "shall supply that which is lacking" (Plato and many modern sexologists), which is paramount to saying that the partner must fulfill or represent the "ego-ideal" which the other party to the contract has constructed as a compensation. The normal child, too, expects from his future, and especially from the one chosen in love the fulfillment of his ideals. But in due course of time, after he has permitted himself to be driven by his "ideal" as a means to an end he is able to detach himself from it, descend to reality and reckon with the demands of reality. Not so with the neurotic. He is unable to change his neurotic perspectives through his own power, he cannot dispense with his principles which have by now become fixed and rigid, he has no longer control over his traits of character. Chained to his "idea" he brings his old prejudices into his love-relations and behaves as though they ought to procure for him not reality but the security of his "idea," the triumph of his strained masculine protest. And soon disillusion makes its appearance. For it is introduced by the neurotic himself as a protective measure, as a security against the prospective derogatory effect of his fictive finale. The disillusionment furnishes the adequate basis for a continuance of the strife against the partner, for a recognition of every opportunity for the degradation of the latter. For these were, after all, the most immediate goals of the old preparatory training.

Unconsciously, the fear of the sexual partner hovers in the soul of the growing neurotic as though he anticipated in the approach of that event the end of his masculine fiction and with it the annihilation of his ego-consciousness, of his guiding star, of his security in the chaos of life. He creates for himself ideals in order to detract from reality. He screws his ego-consciousness, often in a narcissistic manner, as high as possible in order to make every partner appear small by contrast. He surrounds himself with a wall of the most crass egotism in order to furnish the proof of his unfitness to himself and others. He arranges in a neurotic manner doubt, uncertainty, awkwardness, adheres to old faults of childhood and constructs new deficiencies in order to keep himself at a distance. He invents weaknesses, submissiveness, masochistic impulses in order to alarm himself. The power of the sex instinct becomes for him an "overvalued idea" (Wernicke), because he feels its need and apperceives his sexual desire as the superiority of the opposite sex. The neurotic is incapable of love, not because he has repressed his sexuality, but because his rigid predispositions lie in the direction of his fiction, in the line towards power. The neurotic caricatures of Don Juan and Messalina are, notwithstanding their sexuality, neurotic. Those who become inverts and perverts have already escaped the threatening cliffs and seek henceforth to make a virtue of necessity. And where thoughts of incest apparently effect a check on the erotic life, it can be shown that to the neurotic, who constantly fears a decision, this represents a secure refuge, that is, the secure way to the mother or father clothed in a sexual simile.

The flight from the partner, especially the flight from the wife, succeeds better in those neurotics who have early succeeded in finding their way to a profession or who have turned to an artistic vocation. It is true that should they be threatened with a feminine rôle, with defeat, the fear of a decision, of their future, of life, of death may overtake them in the midst of their labors. Frequently, however, some sort of tranquilizing occupation furnishes the neurotics the means securing his ego-consciousness, or his talents, in effecting a formal change in his fiction, furnish him the opportunity to contest for the palm of masculinity in art. It is then not rare that the motive and content of his artistic creations reflect that which has driven him into the security-giving sphere of art, namely, the power of woman and his fear of the wife.

The wonderfully effective charm which many myths, many creations of art and philosophy possess for us, is in line with this; the fault of the woman, the banal "cherchez la femme," in all evils. The thought is expressed in a bizarre manner by Baudelaire, "I can form no idea of a beautiful woman without at the same imagining misfortune connected with her;" mythically and sublimely, in the story of Eve, traces of which have never been missing from poetry. "The Iliad" is built upon this foundation, as well as the "Thousand and One Nights," and if one examines more closely, every great and small artistic creation. What is its leading thought? Nothing less than to win a standpoint in the uncertainties of life, in the conflict with love, in the fear of woman.

Woman as a sphynx, as a demon, as a vampire, as a witch, as a man-murdering horror, as benefactress, in all these pictures is reflected the sexual impulse which has become over-excited by the masculine protest and which have their counterpart in the caricature of woman, in the obscene outpourings of gall, in anecdotes and degrading comparisons.   In the same manner the neurotic, philistine male-consciousness and the desire for superiority forces to those firm convictions which would deny woman equal rights, sometimes even the right to existence.

Another turn which neurotic trains of thought may take in seeking security from woman leads as a natural consequence away from reality and life.   In line with this Schopenhauer was led to a denial of life, the present, all time.   (The preparations for this attitude originated in his unfriendly attitude towards his mother.)   Many patients flee in a somewhat less consistent and methodical manner in their fear of woman, but they constantly hanker after the fulfillment of their fiction in phantasies and dreams which they weave about the future.   Every neurotic shows this trait, wishes to illuminate and investigate the future in order to secure himself in good time.   His cautious and anxious expectation gives the fundamental tone to future events, gray, somber, full of danger.   For they must seem thus to him in order to be effective as incentives. Now he is able to keep the greatest danger in sight, draw the lines of his character-traits and predispositions to the fineness of a hair in order to secure himself adequately. Now he believes to have discovered the road to his goal, and instead of ambition, longing after victory and triumph, honor, elevation, power and admiration, he allows his symptoms to become effective. He experiences under the compulsion of his guiding principle, as a prophetic gift, what sober individuals experience through their foresight and estimation of reality. But with neurotic strivings of "anticipatory thinking," attention approaches problems and arranges them in accordance with the neurotic's antithetical mode of apperception, which values a defeat as death, as inferiority, as effeminacy, and victory as immortality, higher values, masculine triumph, while the hundreds of other possibilities of life are annihilated by withdrawing them from attention. In the same manner the way is entered upon to the anticipation of future triumph and terror as well as an hallucinatory reinforcement for the sake• of security. The psychoses show this trend in a pure manner, melancholia and mania as anticipations of the pure antithesis "above-beneath," dementia præcox, paranoia and cyclothyemia as a mixture.

The recognition and construction of traits of character now follow essentially in strict conformity with the goal-idea. The accentuation of the traits of greed and economy is intended to prevent the abjectness of poverty, pedantry, to assure against difficulties, ethical traits of character, against shame, and all of these against relations of love and marriage, against a subjection to the partner, and at the same time furnish the possibility of an attack upon the partner, an ever ready excuse for his own depreciation of others. The device of the "principle of exclusion," is held in the highest esteem, becomes a religious or proverbial principle of life, of the highest wisdom. The uncertainties of our social system, ethical points of view and the difficulties attendant upon the rearing of children, furnish a welcome excuse for the construction of the boundaries of a natural and reasonable attitude towards life as narrowly as possible, while the obscurity and insolubility of the problems of heredity are distorted in a similar manner in order to justify an unwedded life. Many take refuge in religion, surrender their present life, excite their moral and ascetic instincts in order to become partakers in the happiness, in the triumph in the "beyond." An asexual rôle is arranged and everything becomes a means for the attainment of the heightened ego-consciousness which is rendered possible by the neurotic perspective of life and its experiences. At times security is attained through a want of satisfaction in sexual relations, through a heightening of the disillusionment to a marked degree, a device to which the patient plainly lends his assistance.

It is only another phase of the fear of the partner when the patient brings his predispositions into play against the psychotherapeutist. The neurotic female patient combats the man in the physician at the same time, and seeks to escape his masculine influence which she often apperceives as most terrifying, looking at it as she does from a sexual point of view. The male neurotic secretly seeks to undermine the influence of the psychotherapeutist, which influence he apperceives as sexual superiority, and both conduct themselves during the course of the treatment as they had always conducted themselves whenever compelled to take an active part in life, or whenever confronted by a decision.

At times patients are found whose flight from woman is into the past. It is then that their interest for antiquities, heraldry, dead languages, etc., becomes very acute, and they often become quite skillful in this direction. This skill is absent in those patients who instead turn their attention to grave-yards, death-notices and funerals.

I have already mentioned that the "motive of the fear of woman," is the strongest incentive to art and phantasy. Permit me to quote an abstract from Grillparzer's autobiography, which illuminates much of our thesis.

"Like every well-made man I felt myself attracted by the beautiful half of mankind. I was, however, far too little satisfied with myself to believe myself capable of making deep impressions in a short time. Could it have been the vague conception of the poet or of poetry, or was it the reserve of my nature, which when it does not repel, attracts, because of the spirit of contradiction? I would find myself deeply entangled while I still believed myself to be only at the first advances. This promised both pleasure and pain near at hand, though mostly the latter, because my real efforts had always been to preserve myself in that tranquil state which would not render difficult, or even entirely prevent the approach of my real goddess, art."

When both, artist and neurotic, regard the attraction of woman as menacing, as dangerous, as a compulsion on account of the uncertainty of their triumph, when both regard amorous emotions as a subjection, it is only in conformity with the fundamental disposition that animates both. By which I do not at all intend to deny the realities of these relations. An examination of love, be it ever so sober, reveals a mutual adaptation, a subjection of our will. To put forth, however, special efforts to unearth these, to think of them as something significant and to renounce, for this reason, the pleasurable yielding thereto, reveals unequivocally an unconquerable craving for self-assertion on the part of the person in question, which we have frequently shown to be the neurotic's overcompensation for his neurotic feeling of inferiority. The guiding goal forbids the formation of fitting predispositions, or presents them only in the form of an unmeasurable masochistic exaggeration, which is in turn itself used as a protective measure.

At times this craving for self-assertion seeks other channels as soon as it feels its own libidinous tension as the superior power of the partner. Wishes and efforts then emerge to escape this power through satiety, through orgies. Even castration wishes and intents, and similarly ascetic and repentant practices make their appearance, such as flagellation, etc., incited by the unconquerable craving for security, all in order to win peace from the demon, love. Active, constantly recurring perversions, especially masochistic manifestations, can be explained in no other way. They are an expression of the necessity of convincing one's-self in detail of the sinister strength of the partner, in order to be able to construct out of this conviction of the strength of the other and of one's own weakness an admonishing bugbear.   The real result of this, the neurotic's rectification of boundaries, is a strong deviation from the normal path, which path he fears most of all.   The self-degradation thus arranged now furnishes a stronger stimulus for the masculine protest and enhances it in line with the goal-idea.   "It must be night, where Friedland's stars shine."   Now, after these detours, his efforts are again directed along the paths of his neurotic goal, reveal sadistic admixtures and a strong purification fanaticism in case facts or fancies of a coprophilic nature play a rôle.   Or the patient contends himself to create an appearance of justification for his neurotic detours by means of a struggle against the judgment of others, against the law, or often by having recourse to an unheard of logic, and in this way seeks again to prove his superiority.   Thus it is in the arguments of inverts who in the same manner owe their neurotic deviation from normality to their fear of the opposite sex.

The prestige which it is sought to maintain, the masculine protest is always shoved into the foreground, until the enlightening analysis arrives at that point where in the memories of man the neurotically grouped thoughts come to light, i. e., that it is his inferiority, his underdeveloped genitalia which will hinder him from obtaining victory over woman; in the memories of female patients this place is occupied by the feeling of inferiority, by the neurotic terror of the feminine rôle. Along with these rediscovered trains of thought, which have their origin in the earliest years of childhood, one detects megalomanic ideas often in the shape of narcissism and exhibitionism. They are to be readily understood as preparatory attempts at compensation for the feeling of inferiority, such as are produced by the compulsion of the guiding fiction, as secondary neurotic formations which say, "I want to be a complete man." The change of formula which this thought experiences in girls into the ideal, "I will excel all women" has already been mentioned.

I am able to present some of these relationships in the case of the following female patient. A 19-year-old girl came under my care for depression, suicidal ideas, insomnia and incapacity for work. She had become an artist in order to have a profession. With the exception of indications of hereditary tuberculosis and myopia there were no discoverable bodily symptoms. The relatives described her as formerly an obstinate child who left home because she wished to be self-supporting. Her mother and her only older brother died of tuberculosis.

The commencement of the treatment was very difficult because the patient sat before me showing great indifference and answered none of my questions. Only at times did she express herself with a negative gesture, or answered with, "No."

I began to work cautiously, I explained to her that her indifference is identical with her general derogatory tendency, the same being true of her continued silence in my presence, her negativism, her "No," all of which are part of this derogatory tendency now directed against me. I then endeavor to show her that her conduct indicates her discontent with her feminine rôle against which she seeks to secure herself in this manner. She answers me constantly with, "No," which I disregard as something to be expected and which is directed against me, the male, and proceed. Her depression began during her sojourn at a bathing resort. I now maintain with certainty that something must have happened there which had released this "No," that is to say, something which had brusquely brought to her attention her feminine rôle. Thereupon she related that more than a year ago she had been at another resort where she made the acquaintance of a young man, who was agreeable to her, and that tenderness and kisses had followed. One evening the young man had fallen upon her as though he were insane and tried to approach her in an indecent manner. Whereupon she immediately left the place. I call her attention to the fact that she tore herself away at the moment when the young man wished definitely to force her by his behavior into a feminine rôle and added the remark that she must have undergone a similar experience during the present summer. She thereupon related to me that a guest at the resort whose acquaintance she had made a short time previously, had conducted himself towards her in the same manner as the afore mentioned young man. She left the place just as she had done the previous year.

The "return of the identical" (Nietzsche) leads to the belief that the patient must have had her part in the play since both times she helped herself out of the situation by a neurotic arrangement so as to break off at the same moment. In this connection the patient furnished valuable support in the statement that the kisses exchanged had not irritated her. I showed her that she acquiesced as long as the feminine rôle did not enter the question. I explained to her that her initial courage was the masculine idea of conquest in harmony with her masculine aim. At this stage her insomnia vanished. She communicated this remarkable improvement in her condition with the detracting remark, that now she would like to sleep day and night. Those who, like myself, have learned to recognize the tense aggressiveness of patients during the progress of a psychotherapeutic course of treatment, an aggressiveness which is directed against all superiors, in this instance against the masculine physician, and who have thus sharpened their perception for the manner in which neurotics express themselves, will not misunderstand the expression of our patient. The expression shows distinctly that she has detected the result of the treatment, but that she takes the trouble to detract with a light touch from this result and hence from me. She insinuatingly calls my attention to the fact that one evil has only been replaced by another.

More closely questioned the patient stated that during her four weeks of insomnia she had constantly thought during her wakeful nights how worthless life was. We understand that she did not merely think of it, but had worked at it. Now when the male enemy in the form of the physician, whom she subjects to the same valuation as man generally, confronts her and lays bare her craving for security and thus undermines her effort to gain security by means of her wakefulness, she tries, when forced to sleep, to belittle him by asserting a superfluity of sleep.

Neurotic insomnia is a symbolic attempt to escape from the defenselessness of sleep and to

keep in mind the securities against being underneath. The dream is another form of this effort, equal to a compromise, inasmuch as it covers
as in sleep, the defenselessness and consequent
feeling of inferiority by the masculine protest.
The dream, according to my observation, always
drives towards security and has therefore the
function of forethought. That this is accomplished through the medium of facts from experience is easily comprehensible, and thus it is
that in the dream content and dream thoughts
the defeats which one has experienced come to
light, a circumstance which has led Freud to the
formation of his heuristically valuable but otherwise imperfect and one-sided theory of dreams.

After a prolonged hesitation and after having
her attention called to the negative significance
of her hesitation, the patient brought a few days
later the following dream: *"I was in front of
the 'Steinhoff' (Vienna's great insane asylum).
I hurry past, as I see a dark form within."*

In order to avoid all artificial influencing of
the patient, especially in the interpretation of the
dream, I avoid all explanations of my dream
theory and only refer to the fact that the dream
rouses trains of thoughts which betray again how
the patient tries to secure herself against sleep
which is felt by her to be a defenseless condition,
and which recalls to her her defenselessness in re-

gards to life.   In cases such as the one just given, who wish above all to discuss the fear of the feminine rôle, I indicate that sleep may be felt as a feminine situation.

The figure of speech, "lying in the arms of Morpheus," the frequent sensation of being paralyzed, of being crushed, the analysis of nightmares, etc., and the feminine trends which I am able to discover in all dreams, trends out of which the dream raises itself to the masculine protest, and where furthermore the advent of sleep-banishing consciousness awakens an individual thought-association suggesting a feminine situation, prove with certainty the fact that every dream must reveal a progression from femininity to masculinity.   That not every dream is of such a nature as to convince the beginner of the correctness of my conception, I have already emphasized.   This arises from the fact that in a sketch, and we must regard the dream as such, the sense and meaning of mere traces of ideas must be ferreted out and completed, a thing which is never difficult for the experienced.   I teach the patient that he must regard the dream as he would the sketch of a painting, the details of which he is obliged to fill in according to his impressions.

After this explanation the intelligent patient proceeded unassisted.   "Steinhoff means insane.

This point indicates that I am on the verge of insanity. But I hasten away.   Then what you always tell me occurs to me, I am running away from my feminine rôle.   Hence becoming insane and the feminine rôle are the same thing." I now lead her on to endeavor to force a meaning into the dream, and for this purpose make use of the patient's spirit of rivalry which is known to me, in order to excite her zeal when difficulties present themselves by saying, "But one certainly ought to be able to understand something under that idea."

Patient: "Perhaps that it would be insane to play a feminine rôle?"

I: "That would be an answer to a question. What then must the question have been?"

Patient: "You told me yesterday, I should not be afraid of my feminine rôle."

I: "Therefore an answer directed against me, in line with our conversations, a conflict against the man.   And the black figure?"

Patient: "Perhaps death?"

I: "Try now to fit death into the situation."

This was difficult for the patient, although it is wholly clear that she has taken the fear of death as a figure for her flight from the feminine rôle, in order to present it in a sufficiently strong manner.   The connection of sexuality and death is often spoken of in philosophy and poetry.   The analysis of neurotics often indicate this connection in the sense of an affect-accentuating "conditional proposition."

The sense of the dream is now shown to be an expedient directed against the physician, which with our knowledge of the patient's phantasy-life should be made to read: "It would be insane to submit to a man,—equal to death." But according to her estimation, she had already submitted by the fact that she slept since the beginning of the treatment. This dream therefore revolts against sleep, and her derogatory remark that she would now like to sleep day and night, is in line with this. Therefore the neurotic predispositions of this patient against the possibility of a man winning influence over her is laid bare, and it is shown that the patient acted and dreamed as though she were conscious of her guiding purpose.[1]

This essential predisposition, her tendency to detract, her longing for victory over men and her neurotic craving for security, which stands menacing in the background with the terror of death and insanity, had also caused the development of the neurosis as a strengthened security. Through it the patient is unfitted for life. The

[1] Richard Wagner's genius-like intuition in the song of Erda. "My life is dreaming, my dreaming is thinking, my thinking the control of knowledge."

neurotic apperception, which conjures up a connection between love, insanity and death has
something of the ring of poetry. How firmly
fixed this is in the thoughts of the patient is
shown in her first account: the young man had
fallen upon her as though he were insane.

It is often learned from the anamneses of male
neurotics that they had been under the influence
of a strong woman, mother, teacher, sister, who
therefore, instead of their feminine rôle or in addition thereto, played a masculine one, were
above, and to whom the environment did not
deny recognition, sometimes even disapproba-
tion, showing that they were really regarded as
men. This circumstance also often tends to
strengthen the uncertainty of the neurotically
disposed child, who tries to arrive at a conviction
of his manliness by understanding the sexual differences. Especially when one endeavors to
gain security through knowledge a certain sex
inquisitiveness forces him to constantly seek
visual confirmation of his sexual superiority, a
necessity of obtaining definite knowledge and
full comprehension of the female organs which
approaches the masculine guiding line more
nearly, in proportion as it is created out of preparations for the future.

His pathological uncertainty adheres to the
neurotic as a pretext and confirmation of his

fear of woman even after he is married, so that the expression is often heard, that the feminine sexual apparatus, the condition of virginity, legitimacy of children, fatherhood, is a mystery just as a woman herself is. Along with this desire to obtain satisfaction through visual perception of the female organs, there is at times associated in neurotically disposed children a sort of sinister feeling of danger, as though obscure thoughts arose in the mind of the boy that his future life, his victory or defeat were dependent upon the solution he has reached concerning the sexual question. It is in the nature of things, that frequently the opportunity for this sort of visual confirmation is only offered when the woman occupies a position above the boy. Even this small circumstance forms, as I have repeatedly stated, a figurative representation of the feminine superiority in the phantasy of the neurotic individual who stands in fear of woman. Ganghofer and Stendhal give accounts in the history of their childhood of these terrifying experiences which, it is thought left behind permanent traces. The terror was in itself already a security of the injured masculine prestige, and the exciting scene remained as an admonition, to be understood figuratively, of caution in regard to women. Frequently the derogatory tendency sets in at the point where the superiority of

woman assumes a threatening aspect and leads to
a comparison of male and female advantages and
disadvantages.   The abstract and figurative representation of the inferiority of woman, in
dreams, phantasies, wit and science, frequently
resorts to the mode of expression of a lost member, of supernumerary cavities.   One of my patients who suffered from vertigo had a dream one
time following an unusually stormy scene with
his wife which summarily and essentially brought
about a degradation of his domineering wife.

*"The picture of a birch trunk emerged.   At
one point there was a branch with a round swell-
ing.   There a twig had fallen off and I had the
impression as though this was a female genital
organ."*

I have already discussed such dreams, as have
others also.   To me such dreams represent figuratively the question concerning the differences of
sex, which is answered after the manner of children that the girl is a boy who has been deprived
of the male organ.   The above dream fits into the
psychic situation of the dreamer, inasmuch as it
reveals the thought, "I am a man who has been
deprived of manliness, who is weak and ill, who
is in danger of being under, of falling beneath."
Now he has the basis of operation, he beholds his
prestige diminished and takes breath, for the ef-

fort again to regain power.   The masculine protest now sets in in waking hours as tyranny, outbreaks of rage and acts of infidelity.

It might be mentioned in this connection that
one often hears from neurotics that in moments
of personal danger or when they are threatened
with defeat, they perceive a shortening or con-
traction of the genitals, at times also a feeling of
pain which forcibly impels them to a termination
of the situation.[2]   These phenomena most frequently accompany states of anxiety in high
places where there is fear of falling.   The shortening of the genitals in the bath nearly always
causes a reaction in the neurotic individual.   He
feels out of sorts and at times experiences pressure in the head.

I have already emphasized that homosexuality
as a tendency and behavior is the result of the
fear of the opposite sex.   In addition it may
be briefly mentioned that the over-valuation
of the homosexual partner serves also to raise
the neurotic invert in his own estimation.   In
neuroses homosexuality even when carried into
practice is always found to be a symbol by means
of which it is sought to place the individual's own

---

[2] At times this feeling of pressure extends to the abdomen, to
the breast and cardiac region—or affects only these regions, at
times pollutions take place as reactive symbols of the masculine
goal.

superiority beyond question.   This mechanism is
similar to that of a religious psychosis in which
the nearness of God has the significance of an
elevation.

One of the forms which the fear of woman is
especially likely to take is syphilophobia.   The
train of thought of such phobists (Adler, syphilidophobia, l. c.) is usually the following: They
fear that they will not be able to play a dominating part in regard to woman because of some feeling of inferiority, for which they have ready all
sorts of foundations, at times without conscious
motivation.   In this manner, following the increasing trend to belittle woman, they arrive at
suspicious trains of thought which are to secure them against sexual relations.   Sometimes
woman is a riddle, sometimes a criminal being,
always thinking of adornment and expense and
sexually insatiable.   The suspicions constantly
arise that a girl is only hunting for support, is
bent on capturing the man, is crafty and cunning
and always bent on evil.   These trains of thought
are universal and are found at all periods of history.   They emerge in the most sublime and the
lowest creations of art, have a place in the
thoughts and efforts of the wisest, and create in
man and in society a constant predisposition
which develops suspicious and cautious traits, in
order to always keep in touch with the enemy and

to be in good time for the defense against knavish attacks. It is an error to think that it is only the man who harbors distrust of his sexual partner. The same trait is found also in the woman, often less distinct in character, when fictions of her own strength put a check to the doubt of her own value, but flashing up most strongly, when the feeling of degradation becomes overpowering.

In the disputes of pious savants of the middle ages, questions arose as to whether woman had a soul, whether she was a human being, and the general prevalence of similar thoughts is reflected in the insane burning of witches in the centuries following to which government, church and the blinded populace lent a hand. This detraction from women in hate as well as in love which recurs constantly in Christian, Jewish and Mohammedan religious usages, break out irresistibly in the timorous, uncertain man and so completely fills the world of thought of the neurotic, that the most accentuated trait of character in the neurotic psyche is found to be the tendency to detract from the sexual partner. Thus the outposts which offer security to the ego-consciousness become established and the peculiar play of the neurotic traits of character begins. Continuous testing, feeling, attempts to subjugate, to find fault with and to degrade the partner set in, always favored by the fact that attention and interest is directed to a single purpose, to keep in touch with the enemy and to prevent a surprise. As long as the tendency to detraction with its outward expressions, distrust, fear, jealousy, tyranny exists there is no hope of a cure of the neurotic. As we have seen worthy creations of art and literature which have received recognition on all sides owe their origin to this tendency. From the "Lysistrata" to the "kreuzel writers" leads the same path as from the Gorgo Medusa to the Syphilis fad, which arose before the eyes of Lenans or Ganghofer. The guiding line which prevails in Tolstoi's Kreuzer Sonata and which strives after the degradation of woman was perceptible even in his boyhood when he shoved his future bride out of the window. An old guiding line which is revealed in the myth of the poison-girl [3] of antiquity, in the middle ages and in the beginning of modern times in the fear of witches, demons, vampires and sprites has undergone a change of form and has become the syphilophobia of to-day. Poggio relates of a man who had violated a girl. The girl changed into a devil and vanished with a stench.

All these trains of thought returning in the same manner as they do in the dream and in the

[3] Wilhelm Hertz, "The Myth of the Poison-girl." Abh. d. bayer Akademie der Wissenschaften, 1897.

psyche of the neurotic, reveal the cautious man, doubtful of his manliness, who seeks to secure himself from real life just as much by the setting up of scarecrows as by the fear he has of this life itself, because of the veneration of an ideal.

The bantering note in such an attitude toward woman is of little significance in so far as our view is concerned. It shows moreover an effort to be guilty of no exaggeration, to preserve decorum and to save one's self from ridicule by a spirit of wit. The case is similar to that of Gogol whose strong craving for security is perceptible in every vein of his poetry. In his "Jahrmarkt von Sorotschinsk" [4] he makes a character say, "Lord in heaven, why dost thou punish us poor sinners so? There is already so much trouble, why didst thou also send women into the world?" In the "Dead Souls" of this great poet, who was neurotic during his entire life, suffered from compulsory masturbation and died in a mad house, he makes his hero reflect on seeing a young girl:

"A superb little woman! The best about her is that she seems to have just come out of a boarding school or institute and as yet has none of those special feminine traits that disfigure the whole sex. She is still a pure child, everything about her is straight-forward and simple; she

4 From O. Kaus, "The Case of Gogol," Munchen, Reinhardt, 1912.

speaks from her heart and laughs when she feels like it. All possibilities lie in her nature; she may become a superb creature but she may become a stunted being and that will probably be the result when the aunts and mammas set themselves to educate her. They will stuff her so full of their woman's nonsense in a year that her own father would no longer recognize her. She will acquire a pompous and affected nature, will turn and move and courtesy according to rules learned by heart, rack her brains over the questions, what to say, how much to say, and with whom to speak, and how she shall look at her cavalier, etc., she will constantly be in the greatest anxiety lest she may have spoken some superfluous word, and finally will no longer know what she ought to do and will go wandering through life, a great lie. Fie! the devil!— For the rest I would like to know, of what sort she is!"

CHAPTER IX

UNDER the forms of the neurotic lines of conduct for the purpose of securing the masculine protest, trends of self-execration, self-reproach, self-torture and suicide appear in marked accentuation. Our astonishment loses in force as soon as we see that the whole arrangement of the neurosis follows the trait of self-torture, that the neurosis is a self-torturing expedient whose purpose it is to enhance the feeling of personal esteem. In fact, the first stirrings of the aggressive tendency which is directed against the individual's own person, originate in the child from a situation in which the child through disease, death, shame and all sorts of constructed deficiencies seeks to prepare pain for the parents or to keep himself in their mind. This trait already characterizes the neurotically disposed child who has formed expedients out of the reminiscences of the phenomena of somatic inferiority and out of their significance for the maximation of the ego-con-

412

sciousness, for the purpose of increasing the tenderness and interest of the parents. The developed neurosis builds up these expedients and introduces their activity through a reinforcement of the fiction, as soon as this is demanded by the growing feeling of insecurity. It is well known how strong exacerbations take a hand in this, how the hallucinatory character, the anticipatory force of the neurotic assists in this and how the situation of the attack and the disturbances of health with the resultant dominancy over the environment takes place. Paradoxical as it may seem at first glance the neurotic is only at peace when he has an attack behind him. Janet has already called attention to this fact; I can only add as the basis for it that it is because he has then gained the security of his superiority, if only for a short time.

The trait of character of wishing to excel all others is also contained in the feeling to which the neurotic constantly gives expression, that he excels all others in pain. He uses this conviction because it furnishes him with a basis of operation for feeling himself in opposition to others, for avoiding a decision or for making an attack. Thus it happens also that attacks, pains, or a disease are wished for, when the situation demands it. Sometimes the wish alone serves the purpose of an attack, when as a reminder it already terrifies the environment. For the patient's own psyche it is at times sufficient, as a female patient once told me, if a phantasy is formed as result of which the neurotic suffers pain through the acts of another. This brings about the feeling of suppression or mistreatment, awakens the craving for security and introduces the masculine protest.

The significance of the feeling of guilt, of the conscience and self-reproaches as forms of security-giving fictions has already been described. Not rarely one finds in the psychology of masturbation an admixture of traits of atonement and of a desire to harm, the latter to be likened to an obstinate revolt against the parents, the former as a cheap pretext or sanctimonious act.

The injuring of others through atonement is one of the most subtle expedients of the neurotic, for example when he launches forth in self-curses. Ideas of suicide often reveal the same mechanism, which is clearly seen in joint suicides. When one of my patients was treated by another physician with cold douches for impotence, he expressed the wish "that the physician might tear, injure his genitals." When two years before he suffered great losses in business he wished to commit suicide, although he was still a rich man. The motive force of these execrations (v. Shylock) is neurotic avarice. The analysis

offers a complete explanation.   In order to protect himself from expenses for girls he execrates
himself also when he is obliged to pay physicians'
fees.   This is certainly accompanied by a half
conscious feeling that his wishes need not be absolutely fulfilled.   He execrates especially his
levity for this is the meaning of his self-reproaches and execrations, when he has paid a
large account or ought to pay one.   Then every
small expense disturbs him.

He fears the charm of sexuality.   Even his
own sister he would like to throw into misfortune,
or his sister's daughter, both of whom lived with
him.   At the same time he must have estimated
his execrations as of very little importance or
perhaps even expected the opposite.   This is
shown by the great number of his measures for
security, among which the self-execrations only
played an insignificant part.   He secures himself to a much greater extent through the arrangement of impotence.   Self-detraction and
self-torture our patient constructed in the same
manner as hypochondria, in order to hold before
his eyes the feeling of his own inferiority, to feel
himself too weak, too small, too unworthy.
They appear as hindrances and in this way take
the place of doubts.   Neurotic girls who fear the
man, who do not wish to play a feminine rôle,
worry constantly over their growth of hair, their

birth marks and fear their children might be similarly deformed. In many cases they were homely children or were slighted for a preferred brother when they were small girls. In one of my female patients with a compulsion neurosis, her compulsory thought was revealed as belief in an enlargement of the pores of her skin, to be understood symbolically as a security against the feminine rôle. Another form of self-torture is manifested in the tendency to atonements. They may be recognized as simple cravings for security when it is taken into consideration that these patients seek just as little as those with the allied feeling of remorse for the past, to change or better things in the future.

The symptom clearly aims at the future, and this just as much when it reveals itself as of personal emotion in individual form and conduct as when it is revealed socially in religious performances. As in all forms of craving for security, in this case too, it is not at all excluded that recently experienced evil thoughts and acts come to light. Its purpose is to become effective as a restraining admonition and to serve as proof of the worthy intentions of the one concerned. Not last of all in this self-inspection is the impulse to atonement and the emphasis of inner good qualities wherein the contrast to other people is always thought of, so much so, that the tendency to atonement and remorse at times betrays a strongly antagonistic, intractable, inimical note. The epidemic character of acts of atonement is scarcely ever without this pomp, people vie with each other in crying out, in weeping, in self-torture and contrition.

The possibility therefore of gaining a feeling of superiority by means of fasting and praying, wearing of sack cloth and ashes, etc., will have a charm for weak souls as soon as they have the inclination to appear pious and good, religious and sublime. And asceticism will lead to an elevation when it is felt as a triumph, in my sense, as a masculine protest. That in all this there is only an arbitrary valuation, in which frequently the contrast to otherwise superior people is taken as the point of departure, is revealed in the counterparts to the God fearing type, in atheists, militant free thinkers and iconoclasts who seek to demonstrate their superiority in the same manner as the former. Lichtenberg's expression is to be understood in this sense when he remarks, how rare are the people who live up to the principles of their religion, and how numerous those who fight for them. The conversion from militant free thinking to orthodoxy is not rare as is also not rare the conversion from Epicurianism to Asceticism.

Along with this craving for security by means

of atonement the masculine protest plays a rôle as a guide which should not be underestimated. But one must still keep in sight the building material, the possibilities dormant in the psyche, of which it makes use in order to reach expression. There is no doubt that along with this, acts and thoughts of self-subjection come to light, that is, masochistic elements, which according to our way of looking at the subject are estimated as feminine elements of the masculine psyche. How incompatible these are with the consciousness of mankind and the fact that they constantly demand a change of direction in the masculine protest, that therefore, they are pseudo-masochistic phenomena, is seen from the fact that this subjection is connected with a soaring, an elevation. The lines of force also in this case were from below upwards because the person who has made atonement feels himself elevated or cleansed, he speaks with his God, he comes nearer to him than others, than at other times, and "joy in the kingdom of heaven awaits him."

One of my patients "punished herself" after the death of her mother, 72 years of age, with whom she had always lived at strife and to whom she would have been justified in making reproaches, by deep feelings of remorse because of her indifference for her mother, and by sleeplessness. Her feelings of remorse had the character

of compulsory thoughts and compulsory acts.
The analysis showed that she wished to prove her
moral superiority over a sister. The sister was
married, while our patient was tempted to enter
into a liaison with a married man which experience she felt as a degradation. She was, therefore, according to her own opinion degraded in
contrast to her sister. On the occasion of the
death of her mother the masculine protest gave
rise to a situation which again brought her up-
permost, namely, her stronger grief for the sad
event.

In the history of civilization as in the neurosis,
the tendency to atonement not rarely degener-
ates into scourging, flagellation, etc. From the
confessions of Rousseau and from private communications of healthy as well as neurotic individuals, and furthermore from good observations
of the behavior of children, as for example B.
Asnaurow's, we know that in certain individuals
blows are capable of arousing sexual excitations.
This is the real, somatically perceptible moment
which exists in the makeup of these individuals
and which determines the choice of a particular
form of atonement. Patients have told me that
in their childhood they experienced pleasure from
blows on their buttocks, though it was terrible to
them to be beaten. In the later life of these
neurotics flagellation analogously with masturba-

tion and all other forms of perversions is the visible expression of the fear of the opposite partner. I am indebted to a patient for the following communication. She had come under my care for severe migraine. Several years before the onset of the treatment she was subject to day-phantasies in which she saw herself detected in an act of infidelity and punished by a man to whom she thought herself married but who did not resemble her real husband. As a sequel to this phantasy there followed a severe self-scourging until she fell exhausted. This flagellation brought about intense sexual emotions. The analysis revealed that this woman hated her husband, a neurotic hatred, and in this hatred would have readily committed an act of infidelity in order to humiliate him thereby. Now she has gotten to be too old to be of any worth in sex matters, while in former years she was hindered by the masculine protest. For a short time before she thought of flagellation, she played with phantasies of infidelity, but not without securing herself against a realization. The detection by the husband, the flagellation and consequent auto-erotic gratification, all of this had its origin in the anticipatory craving for security and is but a play of phantasy which emphasizes in an especially strong manner the fear of the man. The substitution of her husband by another is the result of her derogatory tendency and equivalent to her wishes of infidelity, her husband is to be humiliated, another would be preferred in his stead. Continuing, she disavows this plausible assumption through an act of infidelity to this other one. In the course of years she gave up this flagellation. The derogatory tendency, however, is directed more vehemently against her husband as well as against all mankind. She developed migraine as soon as she feared that she was losing hold of her domineering rôle over any one. Her disease succeeded too in enabling her to withdraw completely from society. Within her family circle she was absolute mistress as a result of her illness. She succeeded also in degrading in a large measure her various family physicians, inasmuch as her migraine remained unimproved in spite of all their treatment. Even morphine failed in its effect, and I might recommend that a perverse reaction to this remedy in any case should receive special attention. I mention incidentally, as a supplement to the termination of the treatment that she also placed great obstacles in the way of my form of therapy and for a long time sought to expose me by retaining her pain even when openly flattering me. Patients recover as soon as they understand that this motive of adhering to their disease is for the purpose of humiliating the physician.

Incidentally, I will refer to the fact that according to my experience, "religious insanity," phantasies and hallucinations of God, heaven and the saints, as well as the feeling of being crushed are to be understood as infantile megalomanic ideas of these patients and as an expression of their feeling of superiority over their environment. There is often connected with this a hostile feeling against the environment, as is the case when a catatonic permits himself to be commanded by God to give his attendant a box on the ear or to overturn a bed or a table, or when he tries to compel his Jewish relatives to submit to baptism. The soaring in manics, the dements' grandiose ideas are parallel phenomena and indicate the buried feeling of humiliation which demands over-compensation in the psychosis.[1]

In practice physicians often come across children who aggravate symptoms and simulate in order to escape oppression at the hands of their parents. How closely these phenomena border on unfaithfulness without entirely coinciding with it is self-apparent. Remarkable, however, is the concomitant manifestation of signs of som-

[1] Paul Bjerre ("Zur Radicalbehandlung der chronischen Paranoia," Wien und Leipzig, Deuticke, 1912) was the first to describe in a convincing manner the significance of the masculine protest and of the craving for security in the psychosis.

atic inferiority, as well as the emergence of the neurotic character-development, and hence the neurotic disposition. As examples, three cases of observations of neurotic children are given.

A seven years old girl came under my care for periodical attacks of gastric pain and nausea. We found a frail, poorly developed child who suffered from struma cystica, adenoids and enlarged tonsils. Her voice had a hoarse intonation. Upon inquiry her mother stated that the child often suffered from catarrhal troubles accompanied by a cough, which were unusually protracted, as well as from protracted attacks of dyspepsia. Her present complaint had existed about a half year, without any demonstrable organic affection. Along with this her appetite and bowel functions remained normal. The gastric pains developed since the girl began attending school. Her progress in school was an excellent one, but the teacher had repeatedly expressed wonder over the striking ambitiousness of the child. She was very sensitive about admonitions and felt herself slighted for a sister who was three and one-half years her junior. What especially attracted her mother's attention was a definite lengthening of the clitoris, one of the genital anomalies, the importance of which as a sign of inferiority I have already emphasized here, and which was later on discovered by Bartel and Kyrle and emphasized by them as very characteristic. Her skin was everywhere hypersensitive, and the tickling reflex noticeably accentuated. The child frequently asked to be tickled. The child's anxiousness exceeded the normal. The irregularity of the incisors is to be looked upon as a further indication of a somatic inferiority, which points to a defect of the gastro-intestinal tract. The pharyngeal reflex was definitely exaggerated.

One gains the impression from this ensemble of phenomena, that the reflex activity of the alimentary canal was likewise exaggerated. As a matter of fact the child had vomited frequently during the first three years of her life. The frequent dyspeptic attacks likewise indicate an inferiority of the gastro-intestinal tract. Along with this she had suffered for about a year from eczema of the buttocks,—at the termination of the inferior alimentary canal, with itching which lasted for several months and which was cured by the family physician by means of suggestion and with the assistance of a neutral salve.

The painful pressure in the stomach proved to be a psychic reflex which set in whenever the child feared a humiliation at school or at home.[2]

[2] R. Stern has described similar phenomena, of which we have already spoken frequently in this book, as preactive tensions (präctive Spannungen). According to my conception we are dealing here with a planful, albeit unconscious utilization of reflex

The purpose of this reflex which had been constructed on the basis of somatic inferiority lay in the effort to avoid punishment and to direct the attention of the somewhat harsh mother who preferred the younger girl. After the inner perception of this heightened reflex activity, there was obviously fixation and aggravation as soon as the child sought a guiding idea which she could use for the purpose of maximating her ego-consciousness. On account of the brevity of the treatment I was able to discover no spontaneous expressions of traces of ideas concerning a future gravidity, as the anticipated destiny of a feminine rôle. The attacks vanished after a short time, after I had explained the connection to the child. A dream after one of these attacks points in the above described direction. She dreamed:

"My friend was below. Then we played with each other."

Her friend was a preferred rival in the school. Conflicts often resulted, without blows however. She lived on the floor above and they always played in the apartment of the patient. But the form of expression in the dream she related was sufficiently remarkable. When I asked this intelligent child if one would say "her friend was

irritability of inferior organs, with intelligent reflexes ("Intelligente Reflexe").

below" when the person who related the story
was playing with her, she connected herself immediately, and said "she was with me."   But we
will assume that the form of expression is right
and the accent is on the "below," then behind this
is concealed the thought that the rival was under
the ambitious patient as in a conflict.   "The
friend was below" then means "I was above," a
conception as result of which we are able to define the standpoint of the patient.   The "then"
also points in the same direction.   It only has
meaning when we assume that there is an inter-
val between the two dream pictures, such as perhaps: "I must first be superior to my friend,
then I will play with her."

The history which preceded the attack which
followed furnished a confirmation of our conception.   The game of the two girls was as a rule
playing "father and mother" or "playing doc-
tor."   In the first game there was a quarrel between the two girls as to who should be "father"
until the father finally took a hand and reproached the patient that her companion was always more yielding than she, which was the truth.
The friend thereupon received the part of father.
When the family shortly afterwards seated themselves at the table, the child was seized with an
attack.   She ate nothing and was put to bed
and in fact in her parents' room, where at other

times her other rival slept, her little sister.   The dream now expresses a continuation of the same tendency which was served by the attack and furnishes us a hint concerning the patient's equal valuation of her desire for masculinity and her craving to assert her worth.   The representation of the feminine part as that of the subordinate or the one who is beneath in the word, "under," strengthens this view greatly, but not without giving rise to the suspicion that the patient knows the position during coitus.   She slept before the arrival of the younger sister in her parents' room and even later whenever she was ill.   This suspicion expressed in the presence of the mother remained uncontradicted, but had as result that both the children were kept permanently out of the parents' room.   But here we see again how the character-traits of this child were active in the direction of the masculine protest, functionating as distantly placed outposts whose object it was to secure her at a distance against every analogy, every symbolic experiencing of a female destiny, degradation, minimizing of the ego-consciousness, and furthermore, to protect her from all future misfortune.

A similar affection well known to physicians is the school-nausea and nausea at table or shortly after eating which resembles the above described disease in its psychic constitution in that it rep-

resents an unconscious expedient or one which
has become unconscious for the purpose of avoiding a threatened humiliation and for the purpose
of asserting one's own worth.

A 13 years old boy had shown for the past three
years a remarkable indolence, which prevented
his progress at school, notwithstanding his indis-
putable intelligence. For several months past
he had been manifesting a sort of lamenting habitus which would especially come to light whenever he was admonished for any cause whatever.
His father and mother had probably always been
a little too harsh with him, but as far as I could
obtain information their admonitions only referred to his slowness in eating and dressing and
to his eagerness for reading. Lately things had
come to such a pass that the boy began to cry
whenever he was reminded of anything or when
any one hurried him. The result of this condition was a more cautious attitude on the part of
the parents, though they thought they could not
dispense with admonitions entirely on account of
the sluggishness of the boy.

An inquiry concerning his last fit of weeping
showed that he had been admonished to hurry to
school, after he had been striving for half an
hour before the glass to brush his stubborn hair
smooth. The analysis showed that he saw himself nearing difficulty and wished to secure him-

self against painful humiliations by careful measures. He reproached himself severely with
childish sex indiscretions which he had committed
in company with other boys and girls. Above
all he feared discovery by his parents and this
fear reached an extraordinary degree when one
night during a somnambulistic experience he entered the servant's room and to his great surprise found himself in the morning in the cook's
empty bed. This sleep-walking was, as in all
other cases which I have been able to penetrate,
the result of the masculine protest against the
feeling of humiliation. The day before he was
transferred from the intermediary to the elementary school because of poor progress. The
impression which this scene made upon him was
so great, the fear that he might betray during his
somnambulistic experiences, the secrets between
him and his friends, because like all other som-
nambulists he talked in his sleep, was so terrifying that it led him to very strong measures of
security. The thoughts were first in regard to
his erections which he sought to conceal carefully
from his parents. This he accomplished by a
downward stroking of his erected penis with his
hand. By this time the craving for security had
taken possession of him to such an extent that
he treated the hair which stubbornly persisted in
standing up as if it were a sexual organ, as in

fact the craving for security always reaches beyond what is absolutely necessary. In this case we see the modest beginning of a compulsory act whose mechanism regularly consists in a representation of the masculine protest or in the craving for security directed towards it. The latter becomes the content and motive force of the compulsion neuroses when the masculine protest goes too far and is threatened to fall into femininity through inner contradictions, because the consequences would be a punishment, a degradation or embarrassment. It is then, that the safety device itself seems to be the more masculine, although the alluring feeling of triumph may not be produced. Under certain circumstances however the same results may be attained by a fighting against desire in every form, so that a powerful asceticism is valued as a triumph.

As a matter of fact, ascetic leanings as varieties of self torture, found a place in this boy's craving for security, and this disinclination to eat had for its object analogously to abstinence the checking of his outcropping sexual instincts. The boy who, apart from this, was weak became so reduced that the parents were obliged to interfere. Thus they came upon his craving for security which he had gratified with so much difficulty. Then the psychomotor familiarity with the attacks of the parents led to security through crime as a result of which his value again became enhanced.

His eagerness to read also originated from his craving for security. The insecurity which had seized him at puberty compelled him to seek comfort, instruction and a reassuring fear of disease in the encyclopedia. He was incredibly well read on the problems in question. Once fairly on the way to seek security in books, he overdid the thing because the elder brothers and sisters whom he emulated were remarkable readers, also because he acted against his parents, his oppressors in doing this; and thirdly because he was able to satisfy his original masculine protest in this way and follow the heroes of his books in danger and conflict, which was shown by his choice of reading matter—he preferred Karl May.

The third case was that of an eleven years old boy who suffered from a psychically determined protracted pertussis and who at that time still suffered from enuresis. He was an intractable child who wished to attach his father to himself while he tried to avoid his step-mother as a cruel persecutor. The receptive disposition of the father was manifested in his extreme solicitude during attacks of whooping cough. One morning as the mother again reproached the boy because he had wet his bed, he jumped laughingly out of bed and ran about the room undressed

until the solicitous father with an indignant remark to the mother carried the breathless boy
back to bed.   A severe fit of coughing which re-
sembled whooping cough, from which he had just
recovered, closed this scene and caused a quarrel
between the married couple.   When the boy
again went to bed in the evening, he sprang up in
an excited manner and galloped back and forth
so that he again became breathless.   The meaning of the attack was quite obvious.   The boy
wished to again provoke reproaches against the
step-mother and to draw the father to his side.
A suggestive treatment and an explanation of the
purpose of the attack brought about a cessation
of same, but the pertussis still dragged on for
half a year longer.

Analogous mechanisms are at the foundation
of the idea of suicide.   The deed itself is usually
wrecked on the knowledge of the inner contradictions of this form of the masculine protest.   The
psychic change results from the thought of death,
of non-existence, the humiliating feeling of being
about to become dust, of wholly losing one's personality.   Where there are checks of a religious
nature, they are merely the husks, a recoil as
though this action too were a punishment.
Hamlet, up to our time the model of a person
who doubts of his manliness, of the psychic hermaphrodite, who consciously represents to him-

self in reassuring forethought the limitations of his manly protest, who rebels against his feminine line, and not without evading the dialectical change to the manly line, protects himself from suicide by conjuring up the dreams, "To sleep, perchance to dream, ay there's the rub, for in that sleep of death what dreams may come, when we have shuffled off this mortal coil." In the graveyard scene a real horror was manifested because Yorick's skull was of no more value than the others'.

I have for some time defended the view that suicide is one of the strongest forms of masculine protest and represents a security from humiliation by withdrawal. The cases accessible to me of attempts at suicide have always revealed the neurotic structure in their psyche. Signs of somatic inferiority, feelings of uncertainty and inferiority from childhood, a psychic structure which is felt to be effeminate, and the overtense masculine protest answering to this feeling of effeminacy were manifested in the same manner as in every neurotic. A nearer or more remote example shows the trend. The most powerful psychic hold originates from the thoughts of death in childhood which produce a constant predisposition to suicide by shaping the psychic physiognomy under the influence of the egotistic idea. In the previous history of would-be suicides the same tendencies are fond of trying to attain influence by illness, by attempting or by dwelling on the thoughts of death, dreaming of the mourning of relatives to obtain satisfaction in a situation of humiliation or when there are feelings of despised love. And the idea becomes deed in a similar situation of the reduction of the feeling of self-esteem, as soon as this loss leads to a strong reduction of the worth of life and is able to cause the dialectical change of the masculine idea of suicide to be overlooked in the case of a recent humiliation. Thus we must concede that those writers are correct who see in suicide a process allied to the insane constructions. My studies and those of Bartel's on the inferiority of organ, especially the inferiority of the sexual apparatus, are in harmony with this.

In the neuroses the probability of a correction is stronger, if it does not always prevent suicide. It seems, that the profound consideration of the problem of suicide which with the neurotic usually lasts for years is in itself a sign and at the same time a contributory cause of the correction. And in fact the deeds and thoughts of neurotics are full of thoughts of death. Here is the dream of a neurotic who was under treatment on account of stuttering and psychic impotence, during a night after he had waited in vain for a letter from his bride:

"I thought I was dead. My relatives stood about the coffin and conducted themselves as though they were in despair."

The patient remembered having often had thoughts in childhood that he would like to die because his parents preferred his younger brother. He had always been persecuted by the thought that because of hydrocele and because of smallness of the genital organs he was inferior and would have no children. Later he thought to protect himself by humiliation of women and great distrust of them to protect himself against them and unhappiness in marriage. In reality he felt too weak and was afraid of women. Just as he feared this test in marriage he avoided all decisions through a factor which had become motor. His impotence set in when he received a favorable answer from his bride, as an excuse, an expedient to postpone marriage. In the dream, the thought that his bride might prefer another is reflected. With this was connected an attempt at a solution by means of which he could divert her whole love to himself, in which, as in the arrangement of his impotence the possibility of marriage was eliminated.

CHAPTER X

IN this chapter I will refer to another series of
character-traits displayed by neurotics, such as
are often found in the foreground of psychoanalytic observations where they merely influence
the external picture of the neurosis. They
merely assist in constructing the neurotic indi-
viduality, but just on this account may lend to
the special neurosis a particular direction, or may
provoke a definite fate in the conflict with the
environment. Thus it may happen that the neurotic's *esprit de famille* may be revealed in an
especially obtrusive manner, that genealogical investigations may fill a part of the neurotic's
thinking, which conceals more deeply seated
traits, often of the nature of an unjustifiable
pride of ancestry, which is then utilized as a
striving against the social obligations which go
with sexual relations and marriage, similarly as
the hunting out of heredity of disease is utilized.
This readily succeeds through an arrangement of

extreme affection for certain members of the
family, or for the entire family. This affection
originates from the compulsion of the same guiding fiction with its internal contradiction upon
which the fear of decisions and of the sexual partner rests. This expedient then serves the purpose of gaining mastery over the family circle,
for which purpose the family bond is taken as
something holy. In neurotics the break with the
family borders on the *esprit de famille,* as soon as
the craving for security makes itself felt more
strongly and requires proof that it is impossible
to depend even on blood relations. Misanthropy
as an abstract guiding line and refuge in solitude
are then not rare occurrences and are plainly revealed in the psychosis.

The subordination of the character-traits to
the guiding fiction may be seen especially clearly
in the antithetical traits of refractoriness and
obedience,[1] which singly or intermingled in varying degrees contribute much to the coloring of the
neurotic psyche. Insight into the construction
of these character-traits, which have been ab-
stracted from neutral, actual impressions of the
pre-neurotic period and have then been neurotically grouped and worked over into guiding
lines, teaches us much concerning the origin, the
meaning and purpose of a given character.

[1] Adler, Trotz und Gehorsam, l. c.

The idea of a congenital origin of "character," is untenable because the real substratum for the formation of psychic character and whatever part thereof may be congenital, is metamorphosed under the influence of the guiding idea until this idea is satisfied. Both refractoriness and obedience are only attitudes which reveal to us the jump from the uncertain past into the protecting future, as are all other character-traits.

Timidity as an attitude of the fear of decisions is often accompanied in neurotics by the trait of uncommunicability. These devices work in the manner of an isolation which has for its purpose the withdrawal from the environment of the points of contact. The neurotic who persists in silence sometimes shows his superiority and derogatory tendency also in the rôle of kill-joy, or he arranges through his silence and apparent want of ideas the proof that he is not the equal of others, especially when these are in the majority, and that he is especially unfit for marriage. In the taking up and accentuating the antithesis of the above, loquaciousness, I have at times discovered the proof for the conviction that the individual cannot keep a secret. Another form of attack and detraction is found in the loud, impatient manner which many neurotics have of interrupting others. The object is often more obvious from the circumstance that he introduces every remark with a "No" or a "But" or an "On the contrary."

A trait of character to which the neurosis owes much of its definiteness and significance, which is always present and which, together with refractoriness and negativism, belongs to the strongest forms of expression of the masculine protest, is the tendency to desire to have everything different or turned around. This trait is found in the compensatory efforts as well as in the striving after neurotic expedients, it exists in the disputatiousness and in the neurotic derogatory tendency and possesses an enormous applicability for the conflict with the environment. It is the counterpart of the frequently observed conservative, pedantic nature of the neurotic and like it permits him to confirm his thirst for mastery. The striving for change and revolution is found at the root of the masculine protest, when the latter is constructed according to an antithesis. "The essential of all feminine dialectic is said to be: to wish everything different," announces E. Fuchs in "Die Frau in der Karikatur." In dress, morals, attitude, and movement, something bizarre is always revealed, usually with some pretext. One of my patients often turned herself around in sleep in such a way that when she awoke she found herself lying in the opposite direction. In waking hours also

she sought to turn everything upside down.
One of her favorite phrases was, "On the contrary," as an objection to the opinion of others.
The wish to be above, to ride, to wear the pants
is often found to be expressed in patients of this
sort in an extraordinarily clear manner. In the
psychotherapeutic treatment this trait is manifested from beginning to end, as is the case with
negativism in catatonics, may be always anticipated and extends to the most trivial things.
Very often these neurotic tendencies to contrari-
ness are manifested in the form of a notion that
the physician could come to the patient, not the
patient to the physician. Predictions should as
a rule be avoided in the treatment of neurotics,
but where there is a strong tendency to turn
things around the physician will always be put
in the wrong.

The effort is constantly made to make up-
down; right-left; before-behind, because the guiding fiction demands symbolically the turning
around, that is, the changing from feminine to
masculine. Words and writing are turned
around (mirror writing), morality, sexual conduct, dreams are turned into opposites and follow in reverse sequence and sometimes playfully,
but at other times offensively, thoughts are
turned around. The expedient which is to pre-

serve a masculine line of conduct has accordingly something of the nature of fury.

The application of this "On the contrary" (Umgekehrt) in superstition, perhaps for the purpose of cheating fate by expecting the opposite of what one would like is a frequent trait in neurotics, reveals their complete insecurity, takes us back to the neurotic cautiousness and permits the recognition of the tremendous significance and wide scope which this attains in the psyche of the neurotic.[2]

About this nucleus of cautiousness may be grouped, according to the exactions of the guiding ideal, traits of truthfulness or untruthfulness as the particular situation may demand. They always express the striving after full masculinity, sometimes directly, at other times by circuitous ways. Closely related to these are traits of deception and frankness, the first characteristic originating clearly in a feeling of inferiority, of being under. A strong anticipatory craving for security is revealed by the traits of hypersensitiveness to pain and suffering which keeps the individual as well as the environment reminded that he can only choose those situations in life which can be endured without pain. It goes without saying that the anticipation of labor pains often

2 See also Adler, "Syphilidophobia," l. c.

enters into the construction of this guiding line. The neurotic's phenomena of doubt, of vacillation and of lack of decision which have been so frequently emphasized in this book are related to cautiousness. They always set in when reality influences the guiding fiction in such a manner that contradictions constantly emerge in the latter, when the danger of a defeat, of a loss of prestige, is threatened by reality. There are then, generally speaking, three ways open to the neurotic, which depend upon the strength of the fictitious guiding goal, so that the developed neurosis assumes an aspect in correspondence with one of these. The first way is by fixing the doubt and vacillation as a basis of operation, as is most frequently found in neurasthenics and psychasthenics, the tendency to doubt. The second way leads to the psychosis by means of which under the construction of a feeling of truth,[3] the fiction is hypostasized, deified. The third way leads to a formal change of the fiction under an arrangement of anxiety, weakness, pain, etc., in short to a neurotic, circuitous way in which feminine means are employed to attain the purposes of the masculine protest.

[3] Kanabich, "Zur Pathologie der Intellectuellen Emotionen" ("Psychotherapia," edited by v. N. Wiroboff, Moskau, 1911), approached this thought very closely.

CONCLUSION

OUR study has shown that man's character-traits and their principal function in the life of the individual are manifested as expedients, in the nature of guiding lines for the thinking, feeling, willing, and acting of the human psyche, and that they are brought into stronger relief so soon as the individual strives to escape from the phase of uncertainty to the fulfillment of his fictitious guiding idea. The material for the construction of the character-traits is contained in the psychic totality and congenital differences vanish before the uniform effect of the guiding fiction. Goal and direction, the fictitious purpose of the traits of character may be best recognized in the original, direct, aggressive lines. Want and difficulties of life lead to alterations of character, so that only such constructions find favor as stand in harmony with the individual's ego-idea. In this manner are formed the more cautious, the more hesitating character-traits which show a deviation from the direct line, but examination of which reveals their dependence upon the guiding fiction.

The neuroses and psychoses are attempts at compensation, constructive creations of the psyche which result from the accentuated and too highly placed guiding ideal of the inferior child. The uncertainty of these children in regard to their future and their success in life forces them to stronger efforts and reassurances in their fictitious life plan. The more fixed and rigid their guiding picture, their individual categorical imperative, the more dogmatically they draw the guiding lines of their lives. The more cautiously they proceed in this, the further they weave these threads of thought beyond their own person out into the future and organize on their peripheral ends where contact with the external world is to take place, those traits of character which are required to serve as outposts for their psychic predispositions. With its extraordinary sensitiveness the neurotic trait of character fastens itself to reality in order to change it according to the egoistic ideal, or in order to subject it to the same. Should defeat threaten, the neurotic predispositions and symptoms come into force.

The slight significance of the congenital substratum as far as the formation of character is concerned arises also from the fact that the guiding fiction only collects and unites into a group those psychic elements of which it can make use. It only collects those faculties and memories in

which results are promised for the attainment of
the final goal. In the neurotic reformation of
the psyche the guiding fiction has absolute do-
minion and makes use of experience according
to its own bent, as if the psyche were a motion-
less, concrete mass. It is only when the neurotic
perspective becomes effective, when the neurotic
character and predispositions are fully developed
and the way to the guiding goal is assured that
we recognize the individual as neurotic. It is
then that the neurotic psyche teaches us more
clearly than does the normal that, "Through the
great *being* which surrounds and penetrates us,
there is a great *becoming* which strives toward a
completed *being."* (Durch das grosse Sein, das
uns umgibt und weit in uns hineinreicht, zieht
sich ein grosses Werden, das dem vollendeten
Sein zustrebt.) Thus we find that "character,"
which has found its utility through the guiding
ideal is something like an intelligent pattern
(intelligente Schablone) which is made use of
by the craving for security as well as by the affect
and disease predispositions. It is the task of
comparative individualistic psychology to comprehend the meaning of these models, as Breuer
has begun to understand them in their genetic,
and in our sense, analogical construction, to regard them as a symbol of a life plan, as a simile.
For through the analysis of character by means

of which the line which ever soars toward the guiding ideal may always be followed, we find compressed in one point the past, present, future, and the desired goal.

One will always find that neurotics cling tenaciously to their reassuring ideals. The defense of them becomes accentuated because the patient in abandoning his ideal as well as by a change in direction of his life plan brought about by another anxiously anticipates a defeat, a subordination, an emasculation. The next step in the therapeutic procedure will, according to this, have to be the removal of this strongly antithetical attitude, the resistance of the patient to the physician, and its revelation as a form of the old neurotic ideal, as the exaggerated masculine protest.

Thus as a final word and as an explanation of our standpoint we may sum up as follows: Inferior organs and neurotic phenomena are symbols of formative forces which strive to realize a self-constructed life plan by means of intense efforts and expedients.

AUTHORS' CONTRIBUTIONS REFERRED TO IN THIS BOOK

Studie über Minderwertigkeit von Organen. **Urban u. Schwarzenberg.** Wien u. Berlin, 1907.

Über neurotische Disposition. Jahrbuch, Bleuler-Freud, 1909.

Der Aggressicnstrieb im Leben und in der Neurose. Fortschritte der Medizin. Leipzig, 1908.

Die Bedeutung der Organminderwertigkeitslehre für Philosophie und Psychologie. Vortrag in der Gesellschaft für Philosophie an der Universität in Wien, 1908.

Myelodysplasie oder Organminderwertigkeit? Wiener med. Wochenschrift, 1909.

Der psychische Hermaphroditismus im Leben und in der Neurose. Fortschr. d. Medizin, 1910. Leipzig.

Trotz und Gehorsam. Monatschefte für Padagogik. Wien, 1910.

Die psyche Behandlung der Trigeminusneuralgie. Zentralblatt für Psychoanalyse. Wiesbaden. Bergman, 1910.

Einerlogener Traum. Zentralblatt für Psychoanalyse. Wiesbaden. Bergman, 1910.

Über männliche Einstellung bei weiblichen Neurotikern. Zentralblatt für Psychoanalyse. Wiesbaden. Bergman, 1910.

Beitrag zur Lehre vom Widerstand. Zentralblatt für Psychoanalyse. Wiesbaden. Bergman, 1910.

Syphilidophobie. Zentralblatt für Psychoanalyse. Wiesbaden. Bergman, 1910.

Zur Determination des Charakters. Vortrag, gehalten in der Gesellschaft für Psychologie an der Universität in Wien, 1909.

THE END

INDEX

449

THE END